The Treatment of
**Prostatic Hypertrophy
and Neoplasia**

The Treatment of
Prostatic Hypertrophy and Neoplasia

Edited by
John E. Castro, B.Sc., F.R.C.S., F.R.C.S.E.,
M.S., Ph.D.

MTP
Medical and Technical Publishing Co Ltd

Published by

MTP
MEDICAL AND TECHNICAL
PUBLISHING CO LTD
PO Box 55, St Leonard's House,
St Leonardgate,
Lancaster, Lancs

 ISBN 978-94-015-7192-0   ISBN 978-94-015-7190-6 (eBook)
 DOI 10.1007/978-94-015-7190-6

First published 1974

Filmset by Technical Filmsetters Europe Ltd

Contents

List of Contributors

G. D. Chisholm, Ch.M., F.R.C.S., F.R.C.S.E.
Consultant Urological Surgeon, Hammersmith Hospital and
St Peter's Hospital, London. Senior Lecturer in Urology
Royal Postgraduate Medical School
London W12 0HS, England

R. H. Flocks, M.D.
Professor and Head, Department of Urology
University of Iowa Hospitals
Iowa City, Iowa 52242, USA

L. M. Franks, M.D., F.C.A.P., F.R.C.Path.
Head of the Department of Cellular Pathology
Imperial Cancer Research Fund Laboratories
Lincoln's Inn Fields, London WC2A 3PX, England

Jack Geller, M.D., F.A.C.P.
Associate Adjunct Professor of Medicine
University of California, San Diego
Director of the Training Program in Internal Medicine
Mercy Hospital and Medical Center
4077 Fifth Avenue, San Diego, California 92103, USA

N. Alan Green, M.S., F.R.C.S.
Consultant Urological Surgeon
United Norwich Hospitals
Norwich, Norfolk, England

W. Hendry, Ch.M., F.R.C.S.
Consultant Urologist, St Bartholomew's Hospital, London, and
Senior Lecturer, Institute of Urology, London

J. P. Mitchell, T.D., M.S., F.R.C.S., F.R.C.S.E.
Lecturer in Urology, University of Bristol
Consultant Urological Surgeon to the United Bristol
Hospitals and Southmead General Hospital, Bristol, England

Foreword

In 1963 Professor Huggins[1] wrote "more than one half of the male population over the age of 50 suffer from benign tumors known as prostatic hypertrophy. Often an enlarged prostate is the only difficulty to cloud an otherwise tranquil old age".

This statement emphasizes two important features of benign prostatic hypertrophy (BPH); the frequency with which it occurs and its association with increasing age. The true incidence is difficult to determine as most data relate to selected groups of patients; moreover, the diagnostic criteria of prostatic hypertrophy are not clearly defined. Normality merges imperceptibly into abnormality, for even in men who are clinically normal, rates of urinary flow decrease with increasing age[2].

Despite these inaccuracies, incidence figures show the magnitude of the problem; Flocks (1963)[3] reported that 65% of American men over 60 years suffer from it and in a selected group of Danish men 43% had symptoms of the disease[4]; similar figures are reported for the United Kingdom[5].

At present most patients with BPH, who need treatment, undergo surgical prostatectomy which may be considered the usual treatment. The frequency of the disease alone, creates certain problems, for annually more than 30 000 men are admitted to hospital in the United States with this as a primary diagnosis and with an ageing population the figures can be expected to increase.

The most common age for prostatectomy is the seventh decade[6], so that it is not surprizing that patients needing operation frequently have other medical conditions[7]. Post operative mortality depends upon selection of patients with respect to age and associated medical illnesses; but most surgeons report a mortality rate of about 3%. However, the effect of increasing age is clearly shown in the results described be Watts[6]; in his patients overall mortality was 4·4%; for patients under 80 years of age it was 1·6%, but for those over 80 years it increased to 13·3%.

Untreated BPH is rarely a fatal disease, and operations are undertaken to improve the quality of life. It is against this background that the mortality and morbidity (Chapter 3) of operations must be considered. Refinements of surgical technique cannot be expected markedly to reduce this morbidity and alternative treatments for this essentially benign condition are therefore needed.

Substitution of conventional surgical techniques by newer methods, in an attempt to lessen trauma, is one approach to the problem. Such is the appeal of destroying the prostate gland by cryosurgery (Chapter 4), for it minimizes anesthetic complications and avoids rapid blood loss that may accompany the usual operations. Although useful in a small number of selected patients the exact place of this technique in the surgical treatment of benign prostatic hypertrophy has yet to be established.

The development of a logical basis for the treatment of a disease requires an understanding of its etiology and pathogenesis (Chapter 1). Carleton[8] in 1900 considered the important causes of prostatic hypertrophy to be:

(i)   Perverted sexual acts, habitual sensual indulgencies and unchaste thoughts.
(ii) Imperfectly treated or neglected simple or bacterial posterior urethral inflammation.
(iii) Obstruction in the urethral canal and other structural changes.
(iv) Abnormal functional activity of the testes.

Today the emphasis is on the last of these for there is considerable evidence (Chapters 1 and 2) that testicular steroids have some association with the disease. Based on the hypothesis that BPH results from changes in the secretion of testicular hormones several medical treatments that depend on alteration of the endocrine milieu have been used (Chapter 2). Some of these appear to affect the prostate, but the clinical responses of patients treated in this way do not compare with the results of surgical prostatectomy.

Cancer of the prostate is a common disease. At present, rational selection of the best treatment for an individual patient is difficult for a variety of methods are available and this itself suggests that the optimum treatment has yet to be decided.

When conservative treatments (Chapter 5) are used, the outcome is dictated by the heterogenicity of the cellular population of the tumor. Heterogenicity is important for it will determine the percentage of total tumor cells, which are sensitive to a particular treatment be it endocrine manipulation, cytotoxics or radiotherapy. Non-sensitive cells will eventually cause therapeutic failure and therefore, future developments must allow recognition of the sensitivity of a tumor to a particular type of treatment.

A major point of discussion in the treatment of prostatic cancer is whether to manage early disease by conservative treatments or radical surgery (Chapters 5 and 6). The aim of treatment should be complete clinical cure and whilst radical surgery is the normal approach for this many precedents exist for the use of more conservative methods.

The answer to the best form of treatment will come only by prospective, controlled clinical trials with adequate follow-up. Even then the morbidity resulting from radical surgery might be difficult to quantify.

In assessing the value of major endocrine ablations (Chapter 7) in the management of patients, it is important that objective as well as subjective criteria are used to assess the degree and duration of remission. Because only a relatively small number of patients will respond to these treatments, methods for prediction of the therapeutic response is an important consideration.

Many of the problems of prostatic cancer are common to all malignant tumors. It is to be hoped that with more understanding of the biological nature of malignancy more rational treatments for prostatic cancer will be forthcoming.

REFERENCES

1. Huggins, C. (1963). Introduction, in biology of the prostate and related tissues. Monograph 12, National Cancer Institute, Washington D.C. Government Printing Office
2. von Garretts, B. (1957). Intravesical pressure and urinary flow during micturition in normal subjects. *Acta Chir. Scand.*, **114**, 49
3. Flocks, R. H. (1964). Benign prostatic hypertrophy—the diagnosis and management. *Med. Times.*, **92**, 519
4. Lund, E. (1959). Problems of prostatic hypertrophy in a geriatric department. *Nord. Med.*, **62**, 1784
5. Sandrey, J. (1965). Problems of prostatic hypertrophy in a geriatric department in clinical surgery series. Eds. Rob and Smith, Vol. 6. Genitourinary system, ed. J. D. Fergurson, pp. 372 (London: Butterworths)
6. Watts, H. G. (1968) Prostatectomy: a review of 246 operations. *N.Z. Med. J.*, **67**, 211
7. Erlik, D., Valero, A., Birkhan, J. and Gersh, I. (1968). Prostatic surgery and the cardiovascular patient. *Brit. J. Surgery.*, **40**, 53
8. Carleton, B. G. (1900). A practical treatise on the disorders of the sexual organs of men. (New York: Baericke & Runyon)

1

Biology of the prostate and its tumors

L. M. Franks

Introduction
The development of a logical basis for the treatment of any disease requires a knowledge of the basic factors which initiate the disease process, as well as an appreciation of the structural and functional features of the disease itself. In the prostate we have no firm information on the actual causative agents which induce benign hyperplasia or cancer although we have some knowledge of factors which may influence tumor growth. Some, for example the endocrine environment, can be altered. Others, such as the genetic structure of an individual or race, cannot. Similarly drugs may be expected to cause atrophy of cellular elements in a gland but cannot be expected to stimulate the rapid absorption of muscle and collagen, a process for which there is no normal biological mechanism. In this chapter the basic growth and development of the normal prostate and its tumors will be reviewed.

Prostatic disease has been recognized for very many years — Morgagni[1], for example, clearly recognized the fat, plethoric type of patient likely to suffer from prostatic disease, and described the common site of origin of enlargement of the gland — and in recent years there has been a vast amount of work on the subject but in spite of this many problems in embryology, anatomy, physiology and pathology remain unsolved.

In life the gland is relatively inaccessible, its secretion is difficult to collect, (direct studies of human prostatic fluid can as a rule only be made by collecting the secretion at the urinary meatus after prostatic massage) and it has no known easily measurable function. Consequently most studies of the human prostate must be based on the methods of anatomy and histology. The physiology of the gland has been studied particularly in the dog, largely because a convenient technique

1

for the collection of prostatic secretion from that animal has been devised. The endocrine control of the gland has been studied in the rodent (particularly the rat) and to a much lesser extent in the dog and the monkey. However, the structure of the prostate in these animals differs from that of the human gland and results obtained in these species cannot easily be related to changes which occur in man. Furthermore the two major diseases of the human prostate, benign nodular hyperplasia and carcinoma, do not occur in the usual laboratory animals nor can they be induced in them. A type of benign hyperplasia differing from the human disease does, however, occur in dogs. Prostatic cancer is also seen in this species though rarely. Sticker[2], summarizing his own findings and those recorded in the literature, found 11 cases in 956 carcinomata in dogs. He also reported the finding of 1 carcinoma of prostate in 110 tumors in cattle and 1 among 509 tumors in horses. Engle and Stout[3] (1940) reported a case of prostatic cancer in a very old monkey, and Snell and Stewart[4] (1965) in the female *Mastomys*.

Certain types of prostatic tumors (squamous carcinoma, sarcoma) can be induced by the direct implantation of chemical carcinogens into the prostate of rats[5,6]; in mice[7] and in golden hamsters (Franks, unpublished). Horning[8] has obtained a number of tumors, some squamous, some adenocarcinomatous, in strips of prostatic epithelium which were removed from mice, wrapped round crystals of methylcholanthrene and transplanted subcutaneously into other male mice of the same strain. However, these induced tumors are not strictly comparable with those seen in man.

Morbid anatomical and histological study of human material solves few of the problems of prostatic disease but it allows them to be defined more precisely and some to be interpreted in the light of experimental findings.

The prostate, together with the other accessory sex organs undergoes a series of changes which are associated with the development of, and later decline from sexual maturity. The process of development is uniform in youth and early adult life, but regression is an irregular process affecting different parts of the gland in different ways. There are two main parts in the human prostate, an inner group of sub-mucosal and mucosal glands which may be derived from the Müllerian duct system, and a larger surrounding mass of long branched outer glands (the outer prostate). The so-called lobes of the prostate — anterior, middle, posterior and two lateral — describe only anatomical areas of the gland and seem to have no functional significance. Involutionary changes, at first focal and later involving the whole gland, affect epithelium and stroma of both inner and outer gland groups leading to hyperplasia of the inner group and atrophy which may sometimes be followed by hyperplasia and neoplasia in the outer group. These changes will be discussed under three headings:

1. hyperplasia of the inner group of glands
2. atrophy and hyperplasia in the outer group of glands
3. malignant changes in the prostate

Hyperplasia of the inner group of glands

THE SITE OF ORIGIN OF BENIGN HYPERPLASIA
Benign nodular hyperplasia of the prostate is due to hyperplasia of the inner group of glands. As has already been mentioned, prostatic enlargement in elderly men has been known for many years, but the site of origin of this enlargement was not clearly defined until the end of the nineteenth century. In 1894, Jores[9] described groups of submucosal glands on the trigone and vesicle and in the urethral walls just below the bladder neck, in the normal prostate. These glands, though few in early life, increase in number with age. Occasionally they may be absent. He also showed that some submucosal and median enlargements of the prostate arose from these glands.

Others, however, claimed that the initial change occurred not in the glands but the periglandular stroma near the urethra. He believed that fibromuscular nodules developed in the stroma and that these nodules stimulated epithelial proliferation in the neighboring glands which then penetrated the nodules from the periphery. He showed that many of these fibromyomata contained no epithelium and he correlated the statistics of earlier observers on the frequency of glandular, fibrous and mixed types of prostatic hyperplasia with the inconstancy of distribution of the submucosal glands in the normal prostate. Only when the nodule arose in a gland free area did it remain purely stromal. This theory has been supported in a number of careful papers, e.g. R. A. Moore[10]. My own findings[11] seem to show that both stromal and epithelial hyperplasia, may occur, alone or together, and it is impossible to say that the one occurs before the other. All the tissues of the inner group of glands appear to respond by hyperplasia to the stimulus which causes benign nodular prostatic enlargement.

INCIDENCE AND ETIOLOGY OF BENIGN HYPERPLASIA

Benign nodular hyperplasia is commonly found at autopsy, the incidence increasing with increasing age up to 75–80% of all men over 80 years of age (autopsy cases) yet it has been calculated[10] that only about 4% of men over this age require surgical treatment for urinary obstruction. Thus the urinary obstruction is not due simply to the presence of benign nodular hyperplasia and its exact cause remains unknown. Among the suggested explanations are sexual and alcoholic excesses leading to congestion and swelling of the gland, infarcts which may also lead to an increase in volume of the gland, and involvement or pressure on the urinary sphincter.

Another problem, still unexplained, is the remarkable racial incidence, the condition being very rare in the yellow races. At autopsy Chang and Char[12] found an incidence of 6.6% in Chinese and 47.2% in foreigners. It has been suggested that these findings may be explained by the frequency of liver disease among the Chinese, a characteristic which they share with certain native Africans. Stumpf and Wilens[13] have shown that gross prostatic enlargement is much less common in men over 50 years of age with cirrhosis of the liver than in normal individuals of the same age, and they suggest that this may be due to the failure of the diseased liver to inactivate certain hormones (probably estrogens) which may prevent the development of benign hyperplasia.

There are no reliable figures of the incidence of benign hyperplasia in African negroes, although the disease does occur.

An obvious problem in the investigation of a disease of the elderly in such a society is that only a small proportion survives to reach old age. Although this may be corrected statistically it cannot allow for an element of selection. A less obvious problem is concerned with the social acceptance of illness. This is well illustrated in a series of cases reported from Indonesia by Tan[14]. He showed that prostatic hyperplasia and cancer were present quite frequently in an Indonesian population, although clinical prostatic disease was said to be very rare. In biopsies from 337 patients over 40 years old, prostatic cancers were found in 28, and 55 of 208 patients were found to have benign nodular hyperplasia. Further questioning of these Indonesian patients showed that they did indeed have complaints but they had grown accustomed to their symptoms and had accepted them as a natural thing in their lives. Any interpretation of statistics on the incidence of prostatic disease must therefore be treated with caution and it must take into account factors of this sort in addition to the more obvious causes of under-diagnosis in less prosperous societies.

THE HORMONES AND BENIGN HYPERPLASIA

It has been suggested that benign hyperplasia may be due to hormonal changes associated with aging and in particular to the decrease in androgen secretion which is known to accompany increasing age. Some workers largely as a result of animal experiments consider that although androgen secretion diminishes with age, the secretion of estrogen remains unchanged and that this relative increase in estrogen causes hyperplasia of the inner group of glands. They suggest that this inner group may be derived from the Müllerian duct system and consequently responds to stimulation by female sex hormones. Embryologically, although the prostate is generally thought to be endodermal there is still considerable doubt as to the precise origin of the inner group of prostatic glands[15]. However, other workers, in particular Huggins[16] consider that the tall columnar epithelium of the hyperplastic nodules is an indicator of androgen activity and he feels that nodular hyperplasia due to the fact that the inner gland group has a lower threshold for androgen stimulation than the outer. The inner group becomes hyperplastic because of a 'testicular stimulus, presumably androgen acting over a long period of years on a tissue which . . . has a low threshold to androgens'.

This view receives some support from the low incidence in patients with liver cirrhosis. In these cases there is said to be an increase in circulating estrogens which antagonizes the stimulating effect of androgen. One further point of importance is that the disease has never been found in men castrated early in life or in eunuchs[17] so that the presence of the testicle is necessary for the development of the condition.

The effects of hormones on the normal gland in experimental animals have been studied in considerable detail and there is a vast amount of information available on the structural and biochemical changes induced. These are summarized in a series of reviews, e.g. Price and Williams-Ashman[18], Vollmer[19] and Ofner[20]. Unfortunately there is little information on the changes in man[19]. What information there is is difficult to interpret since most reports are concerned with a description of changes in a limited number of cases.

Attempts to estimate the endocrine status of patients with benign enlargements have also produced confusing results. Most reports, e.g. Marmoston et al.[21] have shown no definite association between the excretion of androgenic and estrogenic steroid metabolites, and benign hyperplasia and Robinson and Thomas[22] failed to show a significant fall in the blood levels of testosterone with aging. Little is known about the levels of other hormones in aging or in benign enlargement. The endocrine aspects of prostatic disease are described in more detail in a later chapter.

STRUCTURAL FEATURES WHICH MAY INFLUENCE TREATMENT

In the established condition a mass of nodules surrounds the urethra and the outer prostate, or the prostate proper, is stretched around the hyperplastic inner glands. The line of separation between the two gland groups is usually quite well defined and in the ordinary operations of subtotal prostatectomy this is the plane of cleavage, leaving the outer prostate behind as the so-called surgical capsule. The histology of the nodules shows a wide range of structure. Epithelia of ducts or acini, or muscular or fibrous stroma in any combination, take part in the process. The hyperplastic collagenous stroma is always the loose, pale-staining stroma propria, i.e. the subepithelial, periductal and periurethral stroma. Hyperplasia is characteristically nodular. The surgically removed prostate generally consists of a mass of such nodules[10,23]. Morphologically, there are five main types of nodule; fibrovascular, fibromuscular, the pure muscular nodule or 'leiomyoma', the fibroadenomatous and the fibromyoadenomatous types in which all elements are involved. The epithelium in the nodules shows a wide range of variation. It may be flat and atrophic, it may be tall columnar and apparently actively secreting, it may be transitional or squamous or it may be a multilayered cuboidal epithelium. Occasionally the hyperplasia may involve myoepithelial cells. Intracystic, fibrous and epithelial papillae are sometimes seen, particularly in dilated ducts near the urethra, and occasionally there may be a peculiar intra-acinar proliferation of spindle cells. Atrophic changes are common in some nodules and similar to those seen in the outer prostatic glands. Cystic change is particularly frequent, the cysts and atrophic acini being lined by a flattened, low, cuboidal epithelium. The stroma of the nodules is made up of interlacing strands of smooth muscle and collagen arranged in much the same way as in the normal prostate. Any treatment, if it is to be successful, must produce its effects on this heterogenous tissue.

The predominant symptom of benign enlargement is urinary obstruction, but it must be remembered that this is not, as a rule, only due to the presence of benign enlargement, which is commonly found at autopsy in patients without any clinical evidence of urological disease. Although benign nodular hyperplasia alone may cause urinary obstruction either by physically obstructing the urethra or by interference with the muscle or nerves supplying the sphincter this is relatively uncommon. If tissue removed at operation from the prostate is examined, some superadded condition, often vascular, is almost invariably found. Infarcts are common, and there may be acute or chronic inflammation or not infrequently quite large and unsuspected areas of carcinoma. Thus the symptoms of benign nodular hyperplasia may be produced by a wide variety of lesions, some of which may be transitory. This makes it extremely difficult to assess the results of treatment in the short term; any improvement may not be a direct consequence of the treatment used. This may help to explain some apparently contradictory results. Good and bad results have been described following almost every type of endocrine treatment. Perhaps the most significant of these is in the series reported by Clarke[24] who found that his best results were achieved by not giving any treatment at all. In the normal experimental animal the epithelium muscle and connective tissue respond in a standard and predictable way to hormones. Androgen depletion, for example, causes atrophy of the whole gland and androgen administration will reverse this atrophy and stimulate secretion by the prostatic epithelium. Similarly the effects produced by other natural or synthetic steroids can be well defined. However, the test animals used are young, and healthy and the cellular response of all elements of the gland is uniform since all are in a normal responsive state. In the aging human male the wide range of cellular patterns found which may range from the actively secretory to the completely atrophic in a single microscope field, indicates that the cellular response in the prostatic epithelium and stroma in these patients is grossly abnormal. In view of the wide range of structures present in the enlarged gland, it seems unlikely that any one drug can produce a sufficient degree of atrophy of all the different types of epithelium, connective tissue and muscle to provide a permanent cure.

At present there seems to be little doubt that the most effective way of relieving obstruction is by the physical removal of the obstructing tissues.

CONCLUSIONS

The cause of benign nodular hyperplasia of the prostate is unknown. The predominant symptom, urinary obstruction, is a consequence of the anatomical location of the enlarged prostate and is usually precipitated by some superadded condition. There is at present no known drug or hormone which will cause a reduction in size of all the cellular constituents of the hyperplastic nodules. Physical removal of obstructing tissue is the most effective method at present available.

Atrophy and hyperplasia in the outer group of glands

Accompanying but not directly associated with hyperplasia of the inner group of glands, a series of changes occurs in the outer gland group. These changes, which involve both epithelium and stroma, begin in adult life, (30 years and upwards), and at first affect only small groups of acini but later may involve whole lobules and sometimes the whole of the gland. Although these changes are originally atrophic some may be followed by hyperplasia or neoplasia. It is important to be aware of these changes since they may in themselves be responsible for urinary symptoms. The changes fall into four different groups.

1. Simple atrophy with or without cyst formation
2. Sclerotic atrophy
3. Post-atrophic hyperplasia
   a. Lobular hyperplasia
   b. Post-sclerotic hyperplasia
4. Secondary hyperplasia.

SIMPLE ATROPHY WITH OR WITHOUT CYST FORMATION

Simple atrophy involves both epithelium and stroma. The lumina of the acini become narrow and slit-like. The epithelial cells lose their secretory activity and become flattened with condensed deeply staining nuclei; the cytoplasm is pale staining. There is fibrous replacement of the muscular stroma and sometimes thickening of the periacinar collagen. These changes are similar to those which occur in the prostate of the castrated animal. The peripheral acini, particularly at the posterolateral angles tend to become cystic and this cystic change may later involve the whole gland.

The cysts are generally lined by atrophic epithelium similar in character to the cells lining the collapsed acini but occasional groups of cells may retain their adult form and apparently are still capable of secretion. The cysts are filled with pale staining (eosinophil) secretion with some swollen vacuolated desquamated epithelial cells not unlike colostrum corpuscles.

The cause of this cystic change is unknown but Huggins[16] has shown that blockage of the ducts with muscle grafts in dogs does not lead to cyst formation. He has also shown that in dogs with cystic enlargement of the prostate the secretion produced is normal but greatly reduced in amount. It seems that duct obstruction alone cannot be responsible for this cystic change and Huggins[16] suggests that it may be due to atrophy of the periacinar muscle which thus cannot completely empty the acini.

In the human prostate the cysts may become very large and the contained fluid may have a very high acid phosphatase content. Simple atrophy is a benign process.

SCLEROTIC ATROPHY

This type of atrophy is first seen at a later age than simple atrophy — 60–65 years according to R. A. Moore[25], but it does occur in younger patients[26]. Unlike simple cystic atrophy which may occur in areas of nodular hyperplasia, sclerotic atrophy is almost invariably confined to the outer prostate. The process may involve single gland lobules or affect most of the outer prostate. If a large area is affected the prostate may be smaller than normal.

Microscopically there is atrophy of the epithelium and considerable thickening of the periacinar collagen although fibroblasts are not as a rule prominent. In the early stages there are often large collections of round cells and histiocytes surrounding the affected ducts and acini. These cells lie outside the thickened bands of collagen. The epithelium becomes lower and is finally shed into the lumen which becomes flattened and elongated and the surrounding collagen becomes hyaline. Eventually the lumen is filled by a loose reticulum containing stellate and fusiform cells with connecting processes. The surrounding band of hyaline collagen can generally still be made out. If the involved acinus contained corpora amylacea these remain, lying in a dense mass of fibrous tissue, without surrounding epithelium.

Moore[25] suggests that sclerotic atrophy is probably an involutionary change similar to that occurring in the uterus. However, it is known that estrogens lead to an accumulation of macrophages and later, fibrosis in the prostates of guinea pigs[27], and many workers have described atrophic epithelial changes in animals following deprivation of testosterone or the administration of estrogens. It is therefore possible that the changes of sclerotic atrophy may be due to an absolute or relative increase in circulating estrogens. However, the almost invariable presence of lymphocyte-like cells suggests that there may be an immunological mechanism involved.

POST-ATROPHIC HYPERPLASIA

In a number of cases the atrophic epithelium of the outer prostate undergoes a series of hyperplastic changes. The reason for this is not known but it seems probable that it may be due to hormonal changes, perhaps involving the adrenal. (Both castration and the administration of estrogens cause enlargement of the adrenal in animals but whether this occurs in man with increasing age remains unknown.) The hyperplasia may involve areas which have undergone either simple or sclerotic atrophy and in both cases there is budding of epithelium from the atrophic acini or ducts.

(a) *Lobular hyperplasia*

This type of hyperplasia which is uncommon, may follow simple atrophy and generally involves the whole gland lobule. A central duct or alveolus, generally elongated and often showing some cystic change, is surrounded by newly formed acini. The picture resembles lobular hyperplasia of the breast very closely. The acini are small, regular and closely packed. The lumina are empty as a rule but sometimes contain a little eosinophil secretion. The epithelium of the small acini is low and uniform and the nucleus, which is ovoid and stains uniformly with hematoxylin, fills the cell almost entirely. The epithelium of the central duct remains low and atrophic. There may be some increase in fibrous tissue in the stroma and often scattered lymphocytic infiltration. The process is regular and each acinus is surrounded by a narrow band of connective tissue.

(b) *Post-sclerotic hyperplasia*

This process resembles lobular hyperplasia but is much more irregular and as a rule involves the terminal acini of the outer prostate. Microscopically the hyperplasia appears to involve the epithelium of an acinus which has undergone sclerotic atrophy. Small groups of these originally atrophic cells proliferate and form a solid bud which grows out into and penetrates the surrounding band of dense sclerotic collagen.

Reticulin stains may show a definite basement membrane around these hyperplastic buds, in which lumina eventually form. On cross-section they appear as a ring of proliferating acini around the original gland. The proliferating acini are made up of a single layer (as a rule) of low cuboidal cells with large hyperchromatic nuclei with a well defined nuclear membrane within which are several prominent chromatin dots. The cytoplasm is scanty and opaque and there is generally no secretory activity. The normal relationship of epithelium to the fibrous and muscular stroma is however lost. The stroma is commonly infiltrated with lymphoid cells.

In some cases the epithelium is taller and the cytoplasm finely reticulated and the cells may show some of the morphological character of small acinar prostatic carcinoma but retain the relatively orderly arrangement of post-sclerotic hyperplasia. Acini of this type may contain the basophil mucoid secretion which is otherwise generally seen only in some prostatic cancers.

Small foci of clear cell small acinar carcinoma are often seen at the margin of these areas.

SECONDARY HYPERPLASIA
This is relatively common and may involve groups of acini, single acini or even part of an acinus or atrophic cyst. The stroma is atrophic but the epithelium in some areas is active — tall columnar cells with eosinophil cytoplasm and large nuclei — with intra-acinar papillae and often some secretion. These areas resemble the normal adult prostate and may be normal residual areas in a prostate which is elsewhere atrophic. This type of change is only casually associated with prostatic cancer.

THE SIGNIFICANCE OF ATROPHY
AND HYPERPLASIA
Simple atrophy with or without cyst formation seems to be a benign process and is probably a result of the diminishing secretion of androgen in the aging male. Similarly secondary hyperplasia is probably best regarded as a residual area of activity in a gland which is elsewhere atrophic. Lobular hyperplasia and post-sclerotic hyperplasia are closely allied conditions and although I have described them separately

there are cases in which it is impossible to decide whether a particular area of hyperplasia falls into one or other group. Post-sclerotic hyperplasia is an irregular process and histologically there seems to be good evidence to show that areas of small acinar carcinoma may develop from it. Lobular hyperplasia on the other hand is an orderly process and I have never seen any transition stages between this type of proliferation and histologically malignant tumors. It is possible that it may be an early stage in the development of post-sclerotic hyperplasia.

There is no clear evidence to show that prostatic cancer is invariably preceded by changes of this type, and we have no definite information on the etiology of any of the changes described. Although endocrine changes may be involved the critical problem is that of localization. The factors which lead to the development of local neoplastic or preneoplastic disease must be cellular, and we have no knowledge of their nature.

Malignant changes in the prostate
As with benign hyperplasia of the prostate, although the pathology of the disease is well established there are many unsolved problems as far as the incidence, etiology and response to treatment are concerned.

BIOLOGICAL ACTIVITY OF PROSTATIC CANCER
Before we can discuss the problem of prostatic cancer we must define our terms. Under the microscope and to the naked eye all cases of prostatic cancer are similar, but biologically — that is in the patient — two types can be distinguished: the active or clinical cancer and the latent or unsuspected cancer. The incidence of clinical cases in the United Kingdom is about 16 per 100000 living. It causes about 7–8% of all tumor deaths in men over 50 years of age. However, if prostate glands are removed at autopsy from patients dying of some other disease, and studied microscopically, histological carcinomas can be found in them very frequently, the incidence increasing rapidly with age. At least 30% of all men over 50 years have these lesions, which are indistinguishable histologically from active clinical cancer yet they have not grown or killed the patient. These are latent or retarded cancers[28,29]. Their

growth rate is very low. Some cases of prostatic cancer diagnosed clinically may be of this biologically latent type. As might be expected these are generally cases in which the tumor is discovered accidentally, e.g. patients with benign prostatic enlargement in whom a carcinoma is discovered histologically after surgical removal of the nodules. The fact that cancers of this type have a long survival period must always be borne in mind, particularly when assessing the results of the treatment.

A distinction must therefore be made between the disease, prostatic cancer, which behaves in the same way as cancer in any other site, and the finding of an area with the histological structure of prostatic cancer. The microscope in this instance gives us no guide to the biological malignancy of the tumor although the other pathological features are similar.

It should be remembered that latency is not a property found only in prostatic tumors, but may also occur in tumors of other organs and in certain experimental animal tumors[29].

The following terms are suggested for the different types of prostatic cancer:

1. *Clinical cancer*
   Any case in which a firm clinical diagnosis of prostatic cancer is made and confirmed by histology should be described as a clinical cancer.

2. *Latent cancer*
   These tumors by definition exist but do not become manifest, i.e. they produce no clinical evidence of disease. They are found *incidentally*.

3. *Occult cancer*
   These tumors manifest themselves by their metastases. The primary tumor remains hidden (occult).

These definitions have no direct relationship to size, growth rate, histological structure, local invasion or distant metastases. They are concentrated only with the method of presentation.

ETIOLOGY AND EPIDEMIOLOGY
There are three etiological factors which seem to be closely associated with prostatic cancer: age, race and the endocrine system.

THE HORMONES AND PROSTATIC CANCER

Since the hormones were first shown to have an effect on the prostate they have usually been considered to play a primary role in prostatic carcinogenesis, although the evidence for this is slight. I think that it is reasonable to assume that the main part played by the hormones is to stimulate the development and maintenance of the prostatic epithelium so that a sufficient number of cells is present in which malignant change can occur. The hormones may play no part in the actual process of carcinogenesis. Once a tumor has developed the neoplastic cells may remain responsive to the factors which control normal growth, provided that the cells still retain these particular normal differentiated characters[30]. It seems to be true that prostatic cancer and benign enlargement do not occur in prepubertal eunuchs or true eunuchoids[17]. A simple explanation for this may be that prostatic epithelium does not develop to any extent in these patients.

There seems to be no direct relationship between steroid hormone levels — estrogens, androgens or adrenal steroids — in the blood or urine, and the development of prostatic cancer[21,22,31]. Pituitary hormones, which may possibly be involved have not been intensively studied mainly because suitable methods have only recently become available. An added drawback to endocrine studies is that most have been carried out after the disease has been diagnosed and it is probable that if there is an endocrine basis, the critical changes may have taken place many years before clinical symptoms appear. All these endocrine studies are based on the assumption that changes occur in the humoral environment, but we must also consider the possibility that there may be a primary cellular change in responsiveness to hormones. A detailed study using modern methods of changes in steroid metabolism by prostatic cells during aging may give useful information.

RACE AND PROSTATIC CANCER

There are two other factors involved in prostatic carcinogenesis — age and race. These have been discussed in detail[13,17,30] The original papers should be consulted.

Even taking possible sources of error into account there seem to be remarkable racial and geographical differences in incidence. It has been recognized for over 40 years that the clinical disease was very rare in the yellow races[32]. Mortality and morbidity data are similar. The only consistent finding is the low incidence in yellow races but there is a remarkable variation in incidence in other races. The highest rate (age adjusted morbidity rate) is that for negroes in one particular area of the United States — Alameda County — of 65.3 while the whites in the same area have a rate of 38.0. The regional variations are even more striking varying from 17.1 for non-Latin Texans to 37.8 for urban inhabitants of Iowa. The extremes in Canada range from 17.0 in Newfoundland to 39.0 in Saskatchewan. In South and Central America, Chile has a rate of 11.3 and Colombia 23.3. Other continents show a similar variation. In Africa the rate varies from 4.4 in Uganda to 29.1 in Rhodesia. There are apparently inexplicable variations such as the rate for Bantu in Cape Province of 19.2 as compared with 9.4 in Bantu in Johannesburg. The rate in Indians (6.5 in Bombay, 9.4 in Natal) is low, as is that in Eastern Europe (e.g. Poland, 4.6–12.8) and Israel (3.1 for non-Jews to 10.8–13.2 for Jews). New Zealand has a consistently high rate — 40.0 for Europeans and 40.3 for Maoris. The Japanese have a consistently low rate (3.2–4.3). There are no comparable figures for China but the rate for Chinese in Singapore is 0.9.

SIGNIFICANCE OF DIFFERENCES IN RACIAL DISTRIBUTION

It is difficult to place any reliance on minor differences but the incidence in yellow races is so greatly and consistently lower than in other groups that it can be confidently accepted, even though more critical studies may introduce minor variations in detail. It seems likely too that the high incidence in some groups of American negroes and in New Zealand can probably be accepted. The significance of lesser differences, e.g. between Eastern and Western Europe is less certain. If the differences are due to environment they should be affected by migration. Unfortunately results at present available are confusing[33]. Prostate cancer incidence in Japanese immigrants to the US rose, but to nowhere near the incidence in Caucasians. There are no figures as yet for descendants of Japanese migrants. The original paper should be consulted for details and for a discussion of the influence of an 'imported environment'.

Other migrants from low incidence areas, particularly from Eastern Europe, also show a rise in incidence[34]. This American experience with migrants and the high incidence in two dissimilar racial groups in New Zealand suggests that possible environmental factors may be concerned. Yet other figures, e.g. from Hawaii where significant environmental factors appear to vary little between the races give a widely varying incidence between the races.

THE EFFECT OF AGE ON TUMOR INCIDENCE

The age-associated incidence of prostatic cancer is established beyond any doubt. It is rare before the age of 50, after which time the incidence increases rapidly until the age of 80. The rate of increase then seems to slow.

Ashley[35] has shown that there is a somewhat similar rate of increase for latent cancer, using four series of cases; one from Germany, two from the United Kingdom and one from Texas. When the data was plotted on a double logarithmic scale there was a straight line relationship between frequency and age, the frequency varying with the 3rd power of the age. When a similar plot was made for clinical cancers a similar relationship was found but the slope was steeper, corresponding to the 7th power of the age. According to the 'multiple hit' theory of carcinogenesis originally proposed by Armitage and Doll[36], Ashley suggests that this supports the idea that latent cancer is the result of smaller number of hits than clinical cancer.

An unexpected finding also suggests that the character of some prostatic tumors in the elderly differ from those in younger men. The older the patient the less likely he is to develop metastases and this is not related to the duration of the disease[37]. Some age-associated factors may therefore influence the growth rate and biological behavior of prostatic cancers, as well as their incidence.

THE SIGNIFICANCE OF
AGE AND RACIAL INCIDENCE

The presence of latent cancers even in low incidence groups suggests that, accepting the multi-stage hypothesis of carcinogenesis, the initiation stage may occur commonly. As Doll suggests[38], the increasing frequency with age may be a direct or indirect consequence of the process of aging. The further development of the neoplastic process may then depend on promoting factors which may be environmental or genetic. The fact that other hormone-related cancers such as breast, ovary and endometrium are also low in Japan[34], does suggest that there may be a possible common genetic basis. This again may be due to differences in the endocrine environment, i.e. hormone secretion pattern, or to differences in cellular responsiveness. Both are well known phenomena in different strains of experimental animals. Although differences in endocrine pattern have been reported in Japanese, there is little information about other low incidence groups.

LOCAL FACTORS
AFFECTING TUMOR PRODUCTION

So far, all the factors I have discussed have been general factors which influence all cells in the gland. But since cancer is a focal disturbance we must also consider cellular factors which influence the development of a tumor in one localized area although admittedly in cells which may have been altered by general factors. Again, we have no real knowledge of possible localizing factors, but there is a suggestion[25,26], that a type of atrophy associated with focal fibrosis may be followed by a precancerous hyperplasia. There is little evidence to incriminate other localizing factors, although many have been suggested.

The pathology of prostatic cancer

There are many reviews on the pathology of prostatic cancer, e.g. [28,39]. The basic facts are well known and I shall indicate only areas of interest.

SITE OF ORIGIN AND ITS CONSEQUENCES

There are two main groups of prostatic glands: inner and outer. Benign enlargement of the prostate arises from the outer glands. There are two main consequences of this. The first is that the disease is very difficult—impossible perhaps—to diagnose in its early stages. It may be present for a considerable time before it involves any structure which may cause symptoms. The second consequence is that invasion of the capsule is common and early and the tumor cells soon involve perineural lymphatics and blood vessels in the periprostatic tissues. The extent of local spread is almost invariably found to be greater than the clinical assessment suggests. Distant spread is equally common and almost invariable in patients dying of the disease. Perhaps one of the best indications is the frequency with which prostatic cancer cells can be found in bone marrow punctures especially in the late stages of the disease[40]. Even in latent cancers vascular and lymphatic involvement is very common.

FACTORS INFLUENCING THE ASSESSMENT OF RESULTS OF TREATMENT

The results of treatment of prostatic cancer must be assessed against the biological and pathological background already discussed. The type of treatment can be decided without great difficulty if all the relevant facts are known. There is a very small group of patients with tumors entirely confined to the gland. It is logical to consider radical surgery for this group. The vast majority of patients must be given some form of general treatment, whether it be hormonal, radiation or other. To decide which form of treatment is best we require a method for assessment. Our first problem is that we do not know at what stage any given tumor is at the time of diagnosis.

Let us assume that a disease has a natural history of 6 years. Patient A by chance or otherwise notices a lump immediately it develops, sees a surgeon and has it removed within the year. Patient B for some reason does not seek treatment until the lump has been present for 3 years. It is then removed. Both die with recurrences after the tumor has been present for 6 years, but the survival period after treatment of Patient A is apparently 5 years, whilst that of Patient B is 3 years, although both have had the same type of tumor and the same type of treatment. This is one possible effect of early diagnosis. If Patient A is treated by an enthusiastic therapist interested in early diagnosis and a particular form of treatment and Patient B by more routine methods, the wrong impression may easily be obtained, particularly if only a small series of cases is studied.

A further problem is that we do not know how any given tumor will behave. We have no way of knowing whether any given tumor has a high or low degree of biological malignancy. Some cases of prostatic cancer diagnosed clinically may be of a biologically latent type. As might be expected, these are often cases in which the cancer is discovered accidentally, e.g. patients with benign enlargement in which a carcinoma is discovered histologically after surgical removal of nodules, or patients in whom a small nodule is found on routine rectal examination. Cancers of this type have a long survival period whatever form of treatment is given.

FACTORS INFLUENCING PROGNOSIS

Obviously it would be of great value if there were features which allowed a distinction to be made between patients with latent or slow growing cancers and those with active clinical disease. Unfortunately there seem to be few absolute prognostic features. In one series[46] two groups of patients were compared. One group lived for more than 5 years and the second for less than 3 years. The structure of the tumor before treatment, i.e. grading, and a wide range of clinical, radiological and biochemical tests were studied but no significant differences between the groups could be found, except that people with metastases tended not to live as long as people without. Even here the finding was not absolute since one of the long survivors had metastases when first seen and lived for nearly 9 years afterwards and 4 others lived for 6–8 years. Although histological grading was not of value in this series others have found it of value as a guide to prognosis[39]. I think that this is true in general terms, i.e. a group of patients with well differentiated tumors will have a better prognosis than a group with anaplastic tumors but it may not give a reliable guide in individual cases.

Vickery and Kerr[41] and Esposti[42] suggests that grading based on cytological criteria might be more valuable than that based on histological appearances. The indisputable features associated with a poor prognosis are penetration of the capsule, and the presence of tumor cells in marrow biopsies[43].

FACTORS INFLUENCING
THE RESPONSE TO TREATMENT

Factors influencing the response to treatment will be discussed in detail in later chapters but there are some general features to be considered particularly in the response to endocrine and perhaps radiation treatment.

THE EFFECTS OF HORMONES
ON PROSTATIC CANCER

The original theoretical basis for the endocrine treatment of prostatic cancer was the fact that the growth and function of the normal gland was dependent on a constant supply of testicular androgen. If this were removed, i.e. by castration, or antagonized by giving estrogen, the prostate atrophied. Huggins[44] therefore suggested that, as many prostatic cancers were well differentiated and resembled normal prostatic cells, they should respond in the same way.

The response of many prostatic cancers to this anti-androgenic treatment is dramatic. Clinically primary and secondary tumors become progressively smaller and some almost disappear. The tumor cells become vacuolated, the nuclei become pyknotic and later there may be replacement fibrosis with tiny clumps of inactive tumor cells lying in dense fibrous tissue. *All grades of tumor cell, from the differentiated to the most anaplastic, seem to respond similarly.*

Those tumors which respond to endocrine treatment are referred to as hormone-sensitive but this term can only be applied to the cells which respond and not to the whole tumor. Even in tumors which show severe degenerative changes a few cells showing no signs of damage can generally be found. Often both primary and secondary tumors respond similarly but in some cases, after prolonged treatment, the primary tumor may still be retarded although metastatic deposits are growing actively. In others the primary tumor and soft tissue secondaries may be inactive while bone deposits grow and ultimately kill the patient. *Hormone sensitivity therefore is not a property of the tumor as a whole but may vary from part to part of the same tumor* (see reference 45 for review).

This underlines another general principle in tumor therapy. Most therapeutic agents like drugs or x-rays do not destroy all the cells in a tumor and the result of treatment is often to leave behind resistant cells which later give rise to recurrences. Whether these resistant cells were present in the tumor from the beginning or are actually produced by treatment is not known. One can kill all the tumor cells as a rule by increasing the dose but the trouble is that the higher dosage generally kills the normal tissues as well. Although endocrine treatment will cause regression for a longer or shorter period in about 80% of cases, most eventually relapse and even after the further removal of most of the known sex hormones by adrenalectomy or hypophysectomy many prostatic cancer cells will continue to grow. These tumors have become hormone independent.

Fifteen years ago I drew some conclusions on the effects of treatment, based on figures reported by McDonald[46]. It would seem from these figures that patients with clinical prostatic cancer can be divided into three groups. The first group — about 70–75% of treated patients and 85% of all the controls — die within 3 years. This includes an estimated 20% of all cases who do not respond to endocrine treatment at all, and die within the first year. After 3 years, the difference in survival between the treated and untreated cases becomes much more marked. By 5 years 25–30% of the treated cases, but only about 5–6% of the controls survive. The second group of patients is this 25% or so, surviving for this period, after treatment and the third the 5–6% remaining without treatment. This last group is of particular interest since there must be some natural mechanism in these cases which retards tumor growth.

Very tentatively, I would suggest that in the great majority of cases — that is, those dying in the first 3 years — the effect of treatment on survival time may be an indirect effect, owing to relief of urinary obstruction, control of infection and so on, without any alteration in the natural history of the cancer itself. This would explain the remarkable similarity of results whatever form of treatment is used. The patients who have survived for more than 3 years may be those who have tumors which have been truly retarded, either by treatment or naturally. Since over 5% of untreated cases will survive for 5 years it is reasonable to suppose that this figure may be subtracted from the 5-year survivals in the treated groups, and to assume that at the most, only 20–25% of cases of prostatic cancer show any definite prolongation of life which may be attributed directly to treatment. These figures are open to criticism in detail but I believe that the general principle is probably true.

It seems possible that the effects of radiation treatment are probably similar in that sensitive cells are destroyed, leaving resistant cells to grow.

THE MECHANISM OF ACTION OF HORMONES ON PROSTATIC CANCER CELLS

Although it seems reasonable to assume that endocrine treatment produces its effects by acting through normal receptor pathways this may not necessarily be true. The changes in hormone levels either by endocrine ablation or by the administration of hormones are on a massive scale when compared with any possible physiological alteration. The fact that either estrogen or androgen treatment may produce a tumor-destructive effect in some cases or that *incomplete* ablation of the pituitary may lead to tumor regression suggest that a non-specific effect may be involved. Other examples of an anomolous response can be found. The lesson to be learnt is that we have no real knowledge of the mechanisms involved.

Summary and conclusions

There are inner and outer gland groups in the human prostate. Prostatic cancer develops from the outer gland group and consequently spreads beyond the prostate at an early stage in the disease.

The biological malignancy of prostatic cancer varies from patient to patient and from part to part of the same tumor. Some tumors remain biologically inactive or latent so that there must be some naturally-occurring factor which controls tumor growth in these cases.

Prostatic cancer patients may be divided into groups which differ in their response to endocrine treatment. These differences in response may be due to changes in the host or in the tumor cells.

The temporary state of tumor retardation or latency follows endocrine treatment — generally anti-androgenic — in about 70–80% of all cases of prostatic cancer, but whatever form of treatment is used, about 75% of all cases die within 3 years. Even in tumors which show a marked response, endocrine treatment does not destroy all tumor cells. *Hormone sensitivity therefore is not a property of the tumor as a whole but may vary from part to part of the same tumor.* We need adequate well controlled clinical trials before we can decide which method of treatment is best but before we can do this satisfactorily we need methods to allow us to assess the stage and biological activity of individual tumors before treatment begins.

We still have no real knowledge of the basic cellular mechanisms involved in the control of the normal, hyperplastic or neoplastic cells by the endocrine system. The reasons for the selective cytotoxic effects of endocrine or radiation treatment are also unknown. Until we have this knowledge any form of treatment must be empirical.

We also have little knowledge of the factors which predispose to or initiate prostatic cancer, so that at this stage, preventive measures are not yet possible.

REFERENCES

1. Morgagni, J. B. (1760). The seats of disease investigated by anatomy. London, *3*, 460, Johnson and Payne
2. Sticker, A. (1902). Ueber den Krebs der Thiere — insbesandere uber die emphaanglichkeit der verschiedene Hausthierarten und uber die Unterschiede des Thier und Menschenkrebses. *Arch. f. Klin. Chir.*, *65*, 616
3. Engle, E. and Stout, A. P. (1940). Spontaneous carcinoma of prostate in a monkey. *Am. J. Cancer*, *39*, 334
4. Snell, K. C. and Stewart, H. L. (1965). Adenocarcinoma and proliferative hyperplasia of the prostate gland in female *Rattus (Mastomys)* natalensis. *J. Nat. Cancer Inst.*, *35*, 7
5. Moore, R. A. and Melchiona, R. H. (1937). Production of tumors of the prostate of the white rat with 1:2-benzpyrene. *Am. J. Cancer*, *30*, 731
6. Dunning, W. F., Curtis, M. R. and Segaloff, A. (1946). Methylcholanthrene squamous cell carcinoma of the rat prostate with skeletal metastases, and failure of the rat liver to respond to the same carcinogen. *Cancer Res.*, *6*, 256
7. Horning, E. S. and Dmochowski, L. (1947). Induction of prostate tumors in mice. *Brit. J. Cancer*, *1*, 59
8. Horning, E. S. (1952) The local action of 20-Methylcholanthrene and sex hormones on prostatic grafts. *Brit. J. Cancer*, *6*, 80

9. Jores, L. (1894). Ueber die Hypertrophie des sogenannten mitteren Lappens der Prostata. *Virchows Archiv.*, *135*, 224

10. Moore, R. A. (1943). Benign hypertrophy of the prostate; a morphological study. *J. Urol.*, *50*, 680

11. Franks, L. M. (1954). Benign nodular hyperplasia of the prostate. *Annals of Royal Coll. Surg.*, *14*, 92

12. Chang, H. L. and Char, G. Y. (1936). Benign hypertrophy of prostate. *Chin. Med. J.*, *50*, 1707

13. Stumpf, H. H. and Wilens, S. L. (1953). Inhibitory effects of portal cirrhosis of liver in prostatic treatment. *Arch. Intern. Med.*, *91*, 304

14. Tan, R. E. (1961). Prostatic disease in Indonesia. *J. Urol.*, *86*, 428

15. Hamilton, W. J., Boyd, J. D. and Mossman, H. W. (1964). *Human Embryology*, Cambridge. (3rd Ed.)

16. Huggins, C. (1947). The etiology of benign prostatic hypertrophy. *Bul. N.Y. Acad. Med.*, *23*, 696

17. Moore, R. A. (1947). In *Endocrinology of Neoplastic Disease.* p. 194. (New York: Oxford University Press)

18. Price, D. and Williams-Ashman, H. G. (1961). The accessory reproductive glands of mammals. In *Sex and Internal Secretions*, pp. 366–448, ed. W. C. Young, (London: Balliere, Tindall and Cox)

19. Vollmer, E. P. and Kauffmann, G. (1963). (eds) Biology of the Prostate and Related Tissues. *Nat. Cancer Inst. Monog.*, *12*, 1

20. Ofner, P. (1968). Effects and metabolism of hormones in normal and neoplastic prostate tissue. *Vitam. and Horm.*, *26*, 237

21. Marmorston, J., Lombardo, L. J., Myers, S. M., Gierson, H., Stern, E. and Hopkins, C. E. (1965). Urinary excretion of neutral 17-ketosteroids and pregnamediol by patients with prostatic cancer and benign prostatic hypertrophy. *J. Urol.*, *93*, 276

22. Robinson, M. R. G. and Thomas, B. S. (1971). Effect of hormonal therapy on plasma testosterone levels in prostatic carcinoma. *Brit. Med. J.*, *4*, 341

23. Franks, L. M. (1969). Pathology of prostatic tumors. *Brit. J. Hosp. Med.*, *i*, 575

24. Clarke, R. (1937). The prostate and the endocrines. A control series. *Brit. J. Urol.*, *9*, 254

25. Moore, R. A. (1935). The evolution and involution of the prostatic gland. *Am. J. Path.*, *12*, 599

26. Franks, L. M. (1954). Atrophy and hyperplasia in the prostate proper. *J. Path. Bact.*, *68*, 617

27. Nicol, T., Helmy, I. D. and Abou Zikry, A. (1952). A histological explanation for the beneficial action of endocrine therapy in carcinoma of the prostate. *Brit. J. Surg.*, *15*

28. Franks, L. M. (1954). Latent Carcinoma. *Annals of Royal Coll. Surg.*, *15*, 236

29. Franks, L. M. (1956). Latency and progression in human tumors. *Lancet*, *2*, 1037

30. Franks, L. M. (1958). Some comments on the long-term results of endocrine treatment of prostatic cancer. *Brit. J. Urol.*, *30*, 383

31. Bulbrook, R. D., Franks, L. M. and Greenwood, F. C. (1959). Hormone excretion in prostatic cancer: the early and later effects of endocrine treatment on urinary estrogens, 17-ketosteroids and 17-ketogenic steroids. *Acta Endocrinol.*, *31*, 481

32. Steiner, P. (1954). Cancer: Race and Geography. (Baltimore: Williams and Wilkins)

33. Haenszel, W. and Kurihara, M. (1968). Studies of Japanese migrants, I. Mortality from cancer and other diseases among Japanese in the United States. *J. Nat Cancer Inst.*, *40*, 43

34. Wynder, E. L., Mabuchi, K., Whitmore, W. K. (1971) Epidemiology of cancer of the prostate. *Cancer*, *28*, 344

35. Ashley, D. J. B. (1965). On the incidence of carcinoma of the prostate. *J. Path. Bact.*, *90*, 217

36. Armitage, P. and Doll, R. (1957). A two-stage theory of carcinogenesis in relation to the age distribution of human cancer. *Brit. J. Cancer*, *11*, 161

37. Franks, L. M. (1956). The spread of prostatic cancer. *J. Path. Bact.*, *72*, 603

38. Doll, R. (1968). The age-distribution of cancer in man. In *Thule International Symposia — Cancer and Ageing*, p. 15. (Stockholm: Nordiska Bokhandelns Forlag.)

39. Franks, L. M. (1967). Recent research on prostatic pathology. *Path. Annual*. Ed. S. C. Sommers. (New York: Appleton-Century-Crofts)

40. Nelson, C. M. K., Boatman, D. L. and Flocks, R. H. (1973). Bone marrow examination in carcinoma of the prostate. *J. Urol.*, in press

41. Vickery, A. L. Jr. and Kerr, W. S. Jr. (1963). Cancer of prostate treated by radical prostatectomy. A clinicopathological survey of 187 cases followed for 10 years. *Cancer*, *16*, 1598

42. Esposti, P. L. (1971). Cytologic malignancy grading of prostatic carcinoma by transrectal aspiration biopsy. *Scand. J. Urol. Nephrol.*, *5*, 199

43. Mechan, D. H., Broun, G. O., Hoover, B. and Storey, G. (1966). Bone marrow findings in carcinoma of the prostate. *J. Urol.*, *95*, 241

44. Huggins, C. and Hodges, C. V. (1941). Studies on prostatic cancer. I. The effect of castration on serum phosphatases in metastatic carcinoma of the prostate. *Cancer Res.*, *1*, 293

45. Franks, L. M. (1960). Estrogen-treated prostatic cancer: the variation in responsiveness of tumor cells. *Cancer* (*N.Y.*), *13*, 490

46. *The Natural History of prostatic cancer — a panel discussion*. In Proc. 3rd Nat. Cancer Cong., Philadelphia: Lippincott, 1957

2

Medical treatment of benign prostatic hypertrophy

Jack Geller

Introduction

PREVALENCE OF BENIGN PROSTATIC HYPERTROPHY

Benign prostatic hypertrophy (BPH) results in clinical symptoms in 65% of males over 60 years of age[1]. Adequate surgical techniques are available for treatment of this disease. However, because the patients are usually older, there is frequently coincidental cardiac, renal, or pulmonary pathology, adding to the risk of the surgical procedure. Medical therapy to allow safe postponement of surgery would be useful. Medical prophylaxis capable of preventing this condition or arresting its progress would be even more desirable.

The development of medical treatment for any disease evolves either from (a) specific understanding of the etiology and pathogenesis which leads to a rational choice of drug, (b) drug trials based on clinically derived theoretical concepts concerning the pathogenesis of disease. If successful, the pharmacologic mechanisms of drug action are then used to deduce the etiology and pathogenesis of the disorder, or (c) serendipity, without either an understanding of the etiology or even a theoretical basis for the use of a particular drug. From the early 1930s, when the first serious trials of medical therapy for BPH began, until the late 1950s, attempts at medical treatment for benign prostatic hypertrophy proceeded along lines that clearly fall into category (b); i.e. drug trials based mostly on the theory that BPH was related to an altered androgen:estrogen ratio. These trials with estrogen, androgen, and mixtures of both did not lead to successful therapy of BPH nor to an understanding of its etiology or pathogenesis. Despite this, there are compelling reasons for thinking that BPH is an endocrinopathy. This concept served as the stimulus

27

for the initial unsuccessful attempts at medical therapy with estrogen and androgen in the past; it continues to dominate current theory and design of clinical trials in the field of medical therapy for BPH.

As so aptly stated by Clarke[2], to ultimately prove that BPH is, in fact, an endocrinopathy, 'Koch's Postulates' of endocrinology must be established. These are, according to Clarke, (a) that an essentially similar disease be produced regularly in suitable animals, either by extirpation of endocrine organs or by replacement endocine therapy; (b) that evidence should be forthcoming of the presence of the corresponding altered level of endocrine function in cases of the disease state in man. As we shall emphasize later, these postulates may be very difficult to establish in the case of BPH because (a) no good animal model for human BPH exists; (b) the possible alteration in endocrine function may not exist in the extracellular fluid but rather in the intracellular compartment which is difficult to sample; and (c) the postulated endocrine abnormality may fluctuate over many years, and sampling of endocrine function at the time of clinical disease may not accurately reflect causal events.

Before presenting the evidence supporting the conclusion that BPH is in fact an endocrinopathy, it should be mentioned that many epidemiologic studies have been done attempting to relate the pathogenesis of BPH to race, marital state, sexual activity, or constitution. There is, in fact, a reported difference in incidence of BPH among Chinese[3], the disease having an incidence of only 6% in males over the age of 40, as compared to the high figure in Caucasian men over 40. No difference between Negroes and whites in regard to occurrence of the disease has been noted[4,5]. The incidence of BPH is apparently as high in Catholic priests as it is in the general population[6], eliminating the role of marital status and sexual activity as important in the etiology.

In short, no epidemiologic studies have supplied any important clues to the etiology of BPH except perhaps for differences in racial or genetic factors.

BPH AS AN ENDOCRINOPATHY
The basis for thinking that BPH is an endocrinopathy is

primarily based on the important role of the testes in the development of the disease. Credit for discovering the dependence of the prostate on testicular function is given to John Hunter[7] who, in 1786, published his *Observations on the gland situated between the rectum and bladder, called vesiculae seminales*, in which he wrote that "the prostate and Cowper's glands, and those of the urethra, which in the perfect male are soft and bulky, with a secretion salt to the taste, in the castrated animal are small, flabby, tough and ligamentous, and have little secretion".

Human clinical evidence

The most important evidence that the testes are essential to the development of BPH comes from the work of Robert Moore[6] who did serial sections of the prostate on 28 patients who were either eunuchs, eunuchoids, or individuals with pituitary infantilism who lost their secondary sexual characteristics before the age of 40 years and lived to be over 45 years of age. Moore could not find a single example of BPH in this group. In the population at large, similar studies would have revealed a 50% incidence of nodular hyperplasia. It is highly unlikely that the absence of the condition in 28 consecutive cases in men over the age of 45 would be a chance observation. Other examples relating the effect of castration on prostates came from reports of eunuchs, for example, the Skoptzys of Russia[8], who were reported to have a smaller than normal prostate and to be singularly lacking in symptoms of BPH. According to local custom, these patients are castrated at age 35.

Even more compelling evidence for the major role of the testes, not only in the development of BPH, but in the maintenance of the disorder, comes from the reports of White[9] and Cabot[10] who separately in the late 1800s reported that surgical castration successfully reduced prostate size in males with BPH in approximately 90% of patients. The operation was abandoned because of the high mortality and the development of the transurethral resection about that time. In a report in 1940 Huggins[11] carefully studied the effect of castration on prostate size and histology in three males. His report demonstrated conclusively that prostate atrophy occurred in one patient 90 days following castration.

ANIMAL STUDIES OF SEX HORMONES

When purified sex hormones became available in the 1930s, numerous biologists began to study the effect of administration of testosterone and estrogen upon prostate size and morphology. The use of testosterone in animals produced larger than normal growth of the prostate, but histologically the prostate showed no pathologic changes similar to the human disease, according to Callow and Deanesly[12]. However, the administration of estrogen in the form of estrone, as described in 1933 by Lacassagne[13], produced considerable growth in the dorsal lobes of the mouse prostate, leading to retention of urine and hydronephrosis. These observations were independently confirmed by many investigators over the next two years, including de Jongh[14], Korenchevsky and Dennison[15], and Burrows and Kennaway[16]. Estrogen administration produced primarily an increase in the fibromuscular stroma in animal prostates as well as metaplastic changes in the epithelium. Lacassagne's findings in the rat were confirmed in the rhesus and macaque monkeys, the dog, the ground squirrel, and the guinea pig. Lacassagne also showed that androgen administration prevented some of the histologic abnormalities produced by estrogen. These animal studies led to the theory that benign enlargement of the human prostate gland might also be the result of excess stimulation of the prostate by an estrogenic substance. Robert Moore[6] has emphasized that no true animal models are known which exhibit the exact histologic changes seen in human BPH. Although there are similarities in some of the estrogen-treated animals, the nodular disease in man has only rarely, if ever, been seen in the dog and not in other animal species, according to Moore, regardless of the endocrine treatment employed. Zuckerman[8] cites the case of a single spontaneous example of enlargement of the dog prostate that resembles closely the estrogen-stimulated dog prostate and also spontaneous human BPH.

**Historical review of theories concerning
hormonal imbalance in BPH and
clinical trials of sex hormones in BPH**

Based primarily upon the studies in animals in the 1920s and 1930s of the biologic effects of estrogen and androgen, there followed a wave of clinical trials in human BPH in the 1930s through 1950s employing either androgen or estrogen or a combination of both to correct a presumed imbalance of these testicular hormones.

Androgen imbalance theory

The idea that androgen deficiency exists in patients with BPH and that androgen therapy, therefore, might be useful for treatment of this disease came from animal studies and from clinical observations. As indicated previously, Lacassagne[13] showed that androgen administration prevented the abnormal histologic changes produced in animal prostates by estrogen. In addition, a number of investigators were impressed by the fact that benign enlargement of the prostate usually begins during a phase that has been called the 'male menopause'; it should be possible, therefore, to correct this condition by administering male hormones. The first attempt at this was actually the work of Niehans, who in 1927 performed the Steinach II operation in which the vas deferens is tied off as a theoretical means of increasing production of male hormone.

Clinical studies of androgen administration

Androgens were administered to patients with benign prostatic hypertrophy by Van Cappellen[17], Morell[18], Schmitz[19], Emmens and Parkes[20], Strohm, Edelson and Merryman[21], Walther and Willoughby[22], and others, and all have reported subjective clinical improvement. However, no objective evidence for reduction of gland size or change of prostate histology was obtained in any of these studies, nor in the histologic studies following androgen administration reported by Moore and McLellan[23], and Heckel[24].

Theory of androgen excess

Lower *et al.*[25], and McCullagh *et al.*[26], originally felt that BPH resulted from a deficiency of a hypothetical testicular hormone, inhibin. They theorized that lack of inhibin resulted in an excess of gonadotropin which, in turn, stimulated excess androgen production by the testes. They administered testicular extracts containing the hypothetical inhibin and claimed subjective improvement in their patients. Chwalla[27] has also championed the theory that androgen excess is present in patients with BPH and is the causal factor in producing the disease. This theory has received little other support in the literature.

Theories regarding estrogen imbalance
The idea that estrogen administration might favorably affect clinical symptoms in patients with BPH provided still another therapeutic approach to the estrogen–androgen imbalance theory of BPH. It was primarily the clinical observations that patients with cirrhosis of the liver, a disease associated clinically with estrogen excess (gynecomastia and testicular atrophy), have a decreased incidence of BPH that provided the rationale for the theoretical usefulness of estrogens in this disease. There are a number of studies in the literature indicating that BPH, both in incidence and magnitude, is diminished in patients with cirrhosis. Stumpf and Wilens[28] reported BPH in 30% of cirrhotic patients as compared to 53% of non-cirrhotic patients. The same authors noted that the magnitude of BPH appeared to be much less among patients with cirrhosis. More recent studies, however, refuted this concept[29]. Clinical trials without objective data, indicating a favorable effect of estrogen in patients with BPH are as follows:

Kahle and Maltry[30] administered diethylstilbestrol and diethylstilbestrol dipropionate to fourteen patients with BPH. They observed a decrease in both the residual urine volume and the size of the prostate by rectal examination in all cases. They claimed reduction in prostate size determined by cystoscopic examination in four patients, and by operation or autopsy in nine others. Accurate evaluation of change in prostatic size, as we shall point out later, is not possible with any of these techniques and largely invalidates the study. There are other anecdotal references to the favorable effects of estrogen by Cook[31] who stated that the "use of diethylstilbestrol for benign prostatic hyperplasia with obstruction is seldom of value but is worthy of a trial in patients who for any reason do not wish an operation or for whom the operative risk is too great. In some instances the administration of this drug has been beneficial". Vernon[32] has also commented that "prostatic hypertrophy in the aged can be successfully controlled by the use of estrogenic hormone". The most recent report of estrogen effects on BPH is that of Roberts[33] who treated 56 patients with estrogen. Roberts did not provide any objective evidence for change in gland size or histology; nor did he measure residual urine or urine flow rates. He claims that most of the patients had subjective relief following estrogen. Some patients, he claimed, even had a prolonged remission following a single intravenous dose of Premarin.

Negative results with estrogen in the treatment of BPH
Heckel[34] reported that estrogen produced vacuolation and degeneration in hyperplastic glandular tissue. Although he noted symptomatic improvement in BPH in patients with mild disease, he did not find any beneficial effect of estrogen in patients with advanced BPH who had elevated residual urines. He did note a decrease in gland size on rectal examination in approximately one-third of the patients.

Embryologic basis for estrogen responsiveness of prostate
Theoretically, the prostate should be susceptible to stimulus from estrogen as well as androgen, since it appears to be an ambisexual organ. BPH in its earliest stages is found in the periurethral tissues proximal to the distal end of the verumontanum. According to Moore, nodular hyperplasia is never observed in the posterior lobe. In pseudohermaphrodites, the structure of the prostate is dependent on the sex of the gonad. If there are ovaries present, the prostate is represented only by the middle and lateral lobes; when both testes are present, the entire male prostate, including the posterior lobe, surrounds the urethra[35]. These observations indicated that the middle and lateral lobes of the prostate constitute an ambisexual organ, while the posterior lobe is a distinctly male structure. Comparison of the distribution of benign hypertrophy in the prostate further indicates that this disease involves the ambisexual part of the prostate; in other words, that part which is sensitive to both androgens and estrogens. Estrogen may actually stimulate the growth of the prostate. Wilkins demonstrates this in a report[36] of a 5½-year old boy with exclusive feminizing effects from a tumor of the adrenal cortex that was associated with significant enlargement of the prostate gland.

Enlargement of the newborn male prostate as a result of maternal estrogen has also been reported.

Estrogen–androgen administration

Bauer[37] administered one part of estrogen and three parts of androgen to patients with early BPH. He claimed clinical improvement and reduction in gland size based on rectal palpation. Kaufman and Goodwin[38] studied the effects of an estrogen–androgen mixture in 44 patients with BPH. They noted subjective improvement and improved voiding based upon urine flowmeter measurements in the majority. Prostatic inflammation and squamous metaplasia of the periurethral epithelium were noted on histologic examination. No predictable change in rectally palpated gland size and no significant alteration of residual urines were noted during therapy. They concluded that this therapy was not useful for prostatic hypertrophy.

In summary, reports of the administration of estrogen, androgen, or a combination of both, in patients with BPH have been conflicting. In almost all of the positive studies, the authors enthusiastically report subjective improvement in a high percentage of patients. Many of these reports have been merely anecdotal. Of greatest importance is the fact that few, if any, acceptable objective criteria or controls were included in most of these studies to support these conclusions. The negative studies, particularly those of Heckel[34] with the administration of estrogen, and Kaufman and Goodwin using combined hormone therapy, have included some acceptable objective criteria such as residual urine measurement and some urine flow rate studies.

There have also been some careful histological studies reported of entire prostates removed at surgery following the administration of either estrogen, androgen, or combinations of both. No evidence of histological atrophy has been noted in any of these studies. We must consider the era of therapy for BPH with estrogen, androgen, or mixtures of both, to be an era of the past with no established clinical value.

Despite these negative studies, the effects of castration, both on the clinical symptoms and histologic characteristics of BPH, as pointed out earlier, remain important clues to the possible endocrine basis for BPH.

CURRENT KNOWLEDGE CONCERNING
ENDOCRINE FUNCTION IN PATIENTS WITH BPH

Studies of the biological effects of estrogen and androgen on the animal prostate and the trials of estrogen and androgen effects in human patients with BPH were done prior to the development of reliable and sensitive hormone assays. Lack of reliable endocrine data, as well as lack of appreciation of the need for adequate controls and objective criteria for drug effects, must be implicated as factors leading to the contradictory clinical hormone trials prior to 1960. Since the early 1960s, highly sensitive and accurate techniques for measuring estrogen and androgen in biologic fluids have become available. These techniques, which now allow testing of many hypotheses regarding the pathogenesis of BPH, were largely developed with the use of radioimmunoassay or competitive protein binding. They now enable one to evaluate precisely endocrine function in patients with BPH.

Prior to the 1960s, the urinary 17-ketosteroid assay was essentially the only variable available for androgen measurements; 17-ketosteroids measure weak or even non-androgens as well as the more potent androgens. The development of specific assays for testosterone in blood and urine during the 1960s made it possible for the first time to evaluate androgen status accurately in patients. It became apparent that changes in levels of circulating or excreted androgens are common in aging males (Table 2.1).

Table 2.1   MEASURES OF TESTICULAR FUNCTION

Testosterone assay	Difference between males <40 and males >60
Production rate — plasma assay	Twice as great in younger than in older males[71]
Production rate — urinary assay	Twice as great in younger than in older males[72]
Plasma testosterone level	Not significantly different[71,73]
Urinary excretion of testosterone glucuronide	Lower in older males[74,75]
Metabolic clearance rate for testosterone	Twice as great in younger than in older males[71,76]

However, it was not until the work of Kaufmann[39] in 1966 that it was definitely shown that androgen levels are, in fact, decreased in BPH patients compared to age-matched controls. In this study, Kaufmann utilized the measurement of urinary testosterone glucuronide, which first was extracted from urine, then separated on thin-layer chromatography, and finally measured spectrophotometrically. This same study of Kaufmann was also the first to report an accurate estimation of estrogen production in patients with BPH as compared with age-matched controls.

Kaufmann found that urinary excretion of estrogen metabolites, estrone, estradiol and estriol were similar in patients with BPH to patients of a similar age without the disorder.

Prior to this report, Segal et al.[40], in 1950 had noted that approximately 50% of elderly males, not separated according to disease category, had significantly higher levels of estrogen than normal young adult males. More recently, Nagai and Longcope[41] showed that estrone, but not estradiol, is increased in older as compared with younger patients. In addition to changes in estrogen and androgen with aging, there is at least one published report indicating a decrease in pituitary LH reserve measured by radioimmunoassay in a small group of elderly males with BPH[42]. No age-matched controls were included in this study.

It has also been suggested that prolactin and/or growth hormone may play an important part in controlling growth of the prostate. Grayhack et al.[43] showed that androgen administration to hypoxed rats, as compared to castrates, did not repair prostate weight. In addition, Asano[44] has noted the potentiating effect of prolactin on prostate growth when given in conjunction with androgens to rats. Prolactin effects in human BPH have not been studied.

During the past decade, a new dimension in the understanding of hormone function and regulation has been added. This refers to the measurement of intracellular levels, made available by the use of radioimmunoassay or protein binding techniques which allow the measurement within subcellular compartments of nanogram amounts of steroid and protein hormones. It has now become obvious that the androgen target organ growth cannot be studied by measuring circulating hormone alone. The concept of sex hormone function must now be extended to include the measurement and protein binding characteristics of intracellular hormones, since sex steroid target organs are able to concentrate sex steroids and convert them into active metabolites not present in appreciable amounts in extracellular fluids.

Androgen—Intracellular Mechanism of Action

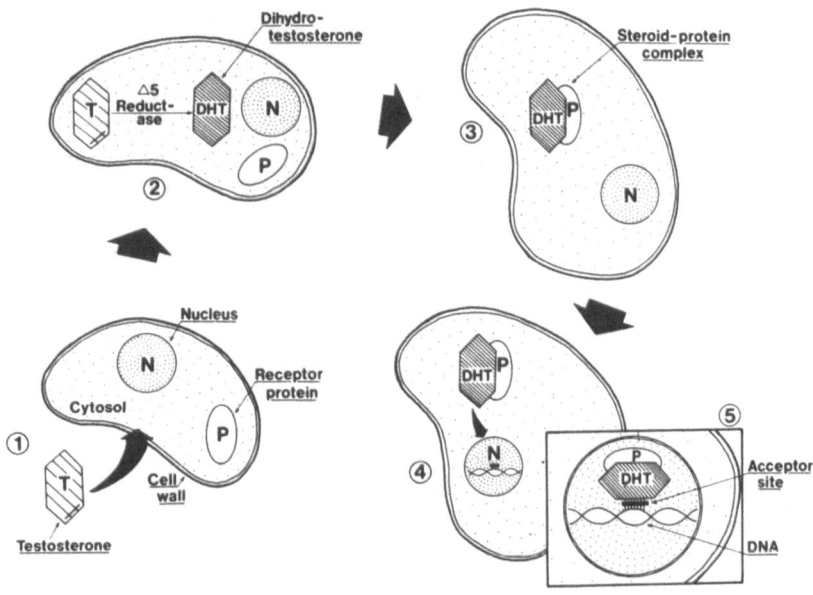

Figure 2.1 Schematic representation of biochemical events mediating biologic effects of testosterone on prostate cells

(1) Testosterone from plasma enters the prostate cell, probably by passive diffusion

(2) On entry into the cell, testosterone is reduced to dihydrotestosterone by Δ-5 reductase in the cytosol

(3) 5α DHT is bound selectively to a specific cytosol macromolecular protein

(4) The steroid-protein complex enters the nucleus

(5) The steroid-protein complex within the nucleus is bound to an acceptor protein where it presumably influences the transcription phase of protein synthesis

The best example of this is found in studies of the rat prostate by Fang[45] and others which demonstrate that testosterone is metabolized to dihydrotestosterone (DHT) within the prostate cytosol (Figure 2.1). DHT, in turn, is selectively bound to a specific cytosol protein, and this complex is then bound to a specific nuclear acceptor. Within the nucleus, the DHT-protein complex presumably affects DNA-dependent protein synthesis and thus cell growth. In animal studies, DHT appears to be the major androgen metabolite present in prostate cytosol and nuclei, while present in only trace amounts in the extracellular fluid compartment.

In the human, very little data is available on hormonal changes within the prostate of patients with BPH. In twelve patients with BPH reported by Siiteri et al.[46], the prostate contained six times as much DHT as was present in the prostate of young normal male controls. This important finding needs confirmation. It points up the importance of intracellular compartment measurements, since no hint of this finding comes from measurements in the extracellular compartment.

The current era of research on the etiology and pathogenesis of BPH

The current era of medical therapy for BPH was begun by Geller[47] in 1964, who reported the effects of 'medical castration' for control of BPH. Based upon the surgical castration studies of Cabot[10], White[9], and Huggins[11], Geller theorized that a non-estrogenic, non-androgenic substance which could suppress testicular function might produce prostate atrophy by medical castration. It was felt to be important in this theory that the substance employed should be neither estrogenic nor androgenic. Both these hormones had been clinically ineffective in controlling BPH, and actually were implicated as possible causative agents in BPH. Since the original report by Geller, encouraging results have been reported with the use of eight different progestational anti-androgens in patients with BPH (Table 2.2).

Effects of progestational anti-androgens on endocrine function in the human

The progestational anti-androgen drugs studied to date in humans effectively decrease circulating testosterone levels. At least one of these agents also decreases estrogen production, thus satisfying the criteria for medical castration. Geller[48] and Scott[49] have both indicated that cyproterone acetate decreases circulating testosterone. Fishman and Geller[50] have also indicated that this drug reduces estrogen production rates in the male to castrate levels, either by direct effect on estrogen production or indirectly by decreasing androgen production.

Cyproterone acetate also inhibits growth hormone release and suppresses the LH rise following clomiphene citrate in human males[51]. Fang[45] has reported that cyproterone acetate in the rat prostate specifically blocks the steroid-protein binding in both cytosol and nucleus. Recently, this has been shown in the human prostate by Hansson[52]; Geller has confirmed this (Figure 2.2) in unpublished data with a more reliable technique which eliminates any possible contamination from testosterone-estrogen binding globulin (TeBG). Thus, at least one anti-androgen studied in humans, cyproterone acetate, not only produces medical castration in the classical sense with a decrease in circulating androgen and estrogen, but blocks intracellular androgen binding. No studies have been done with anti-androgens on the effect of these drugs on the prostatic level of DHT, which, according to Siiteri et al.[46], is increased six-fold in patients with BPH.

Geller has also demonstrated significant decreases in plasma or urine testosterone glucuronide levels following the administration of three other anti-androgens. These include Delalutin, Chlormadinone acetate, and pH-218. It would appear that decreased androgen production is a property shared by all anti-androgens to date.

Cyproterone acetate has also been reported to reduce the content of total labelled radiosteroid in the rat prostate following administration of H^3T [53]. No similar studies have been reported in the human.

Nothing is known about the effects of anti-androgens on estrogen metabolism within the human prostate. That estrogen within the prostate may be important is indicated by *in vitro* studies in which it has been shown that the prostate can convert androgen to estrogen[54]. It has also been shown by Acevedo and Goldzieher[55] that the prostate has enzymes capable of interconverting estradiol to other estrogen metabolites.

Table 2.2 REPORTS OF CLINICAL TRIALS OF PROGESTATIONAL ANTI-ANDROGENS IN PATIENTS WITH BPH

Drug and dosage	Author	Clinical effect of drug	Number patients treated	Average follow-up (months)	Accepted objective criteria employed	Controls	Double-blind technique
Delalutin (17α-hydroxy-progesterone caproate) 3 g/week	Geller et al.[61]	Favorable	8	21	R, V	Yes	No
Delalutin 2.5 g/week	Weinberg[62]	No effect	15	8	None	No	No
Delalutin 2.5 g/week	Jacobs et al.[63]	No effect	20	3	R? Data incomplete	No	No
19 Nor-Delalutin (17α-hydroxy-19-nor-progesterone caproate) 300 mg/week	Nuri[66]	Favorable	41	3	R	No	No
19 Nor-Delalutin 300 mg/week	Crooks[64]	Favorable	7	3	UF	No	No
19 Nor-Delalutin	Vahlensieck[65]	Favorable	5	3	R	No	No
Chlormadinone acetate (6α-chloro-Δ6-17α-acetoxy-progesterone) 100 mg/day	Geller[61]	Favorable	3	16	R, V Study too small	No	No

Drug	Reference	Effect					
Cyproterone acetate (1,2α-methylene-6-chloro-Δ4,6-17α-hydroxy-progesterone acetate) 50 mg/day	Scott and Wade[49]	Favorable	13	15	R, UF	No	No
Cyproterone acetate 100 mg/day	Vahlensieck[65]	Favorable	12	3	R	No	No
Medrogestone (6,17 dimethyl-Δ4,6-progesterone) 100 mg/day	Rangno et al.[68]	Favorable	24	12	R	Yes	Yes
Megestrol acetate (6-dehydro-6-methyl-17α-acetoxy-progesterone) 20–30 mg/day	Lebech et al.[67]	Favorable	15	10	R, UF	No	No
Norlutin (17α-ethynyl-19-nor-testosterone) 5 mg/day	Wolf et al.[58]	No effect	18	6	R, UF	Yes	No
Primolut-Nor (17α ethynyl-19 nor-progesterone)	Vahlensieck[65]	Favorable	19	4.5	R	No	No

R = Residual urine
V = Ability to void
UF = Urine flow rate

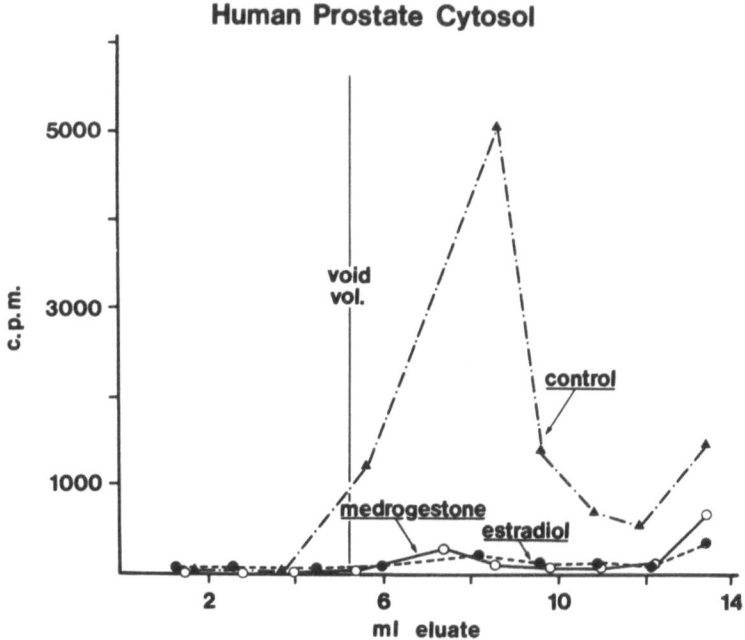

Figure 2.2 Effect of anti-androgen and estrogen on steroid-protein binding in human prostate cytosol

Cytosol obtained from human prostates was precipitated at 33% ammonium sulfate. The precipitate was redissolved in buffer 0.32 M, 1.0 mM magnesium chloride, 0.2 M Tris to pH 7.4) and 10% glycerol, and the redissolved material filtered on G-50 Sephadex. The elution volume in ml is shown on the abscissa in relation to the counts per minute seen on the ordinate. All three curves are corrected to the same protein concentration

In rat studies of Fang[45] and Unhjem *et al.*[56], the binding of steroid metabolites to specific cytosol and nuclear proteins represented a crucial step in the biological action of androgens. If, indeed, the binding of intracellular DHT to specific receptor proteins is important to the perpetuation of the human nodular prostatic hyperplasia, then anti-androgens should be ideally suited for treatment of BPH. Such conclusions are not warranted at this time in the human, since human data concerning steroid–protein binding in cytosol and nucleus is very incomplete.

In the rat, it is seen that the growth and maintenance of the prostate depend upon the integrity of DHT binding to a specific cytosol 'beta' protein*, because no steroids other than DHT, including testosterone and estrogen, compete effectively for the 'beta' protein except anti-androgens. Thus, in the rat, anti-androgens produce prostate atrophy, and this correlates with the specific effects on decreased DHT-protein complex formation in cytosol and nucleus. However, as mentioned previously, the rat prostate may not be a valid model for human BPH. That the androgen steroid–protein binding may not be crucial to the etiology and pathogenesis of human BPH is suggested by the fact that estrogen, which does not favorably influence BPH clinically, can inhibit specific cytosol and nuclear androgen–protein binding *in vitro* in the human prostate. These latter studies were done by incubating estradiol-17β and H^{3}T with human prostate minces in amounts similar to those used for studies of an anti-androgen, medrogestone.

The similarity of estrogen biochemical activity to that of anti-androgen, as regards inhibition of steroid–protein binding intracellularly in the prostate, contrasts with the difference in the clinical effects of estrogen versus anti-androgens, as indicated by a summary of the clinical literature (Table 2.2). This contrast points up the difficulty in linking the molecular biochemical steps in the pathway of androgen action to the pathogenesis of BPH. It is interesting that many anti-androgens also possess anti-estrogen activity in animal studies. Such effects, if they occur in humans, may explain the favorable influence and possibly the mechanism of action of so-called progestational anti-androgens in BPH.

Critique of clinical studies of progestational anti-androgens in patients with BPH

Before critically evaluating individual clinical reports of the effect of progestational anti-androgens on the clinical symptoms of BPH, let us review the suitability of criteria used to evaluate possible drug-induced changes in the clinical symptoms of BPH.

* Cytosol 'beta' protein refers to cytosol fraction precipitating at 40% $(NH_4)_2SO_4$, first described by Liao.

EVALUATION OF CRITERIA
FOR EFFECT OF DRUGS IN BPH

(1) If subjective clinical symptoms of BPH, including frequency, nocturia, urgency, hesitancy, dribbling and strength of urinary stream are used to evaluate the drug effect, then studies must either be carried out for a period of three or more years, or suitable controls must be included and double-blind technique employed with a follow-up for six or more months. The need for such criteria is based upon the natural history of BPH which, as pointed out by Clarke[2] in 1937, indicates that improvement lasting approximately three years in clinical symptoms of prostatism occurred in 60% of patients with mild-to-moderate BPH who were followed without specific therapy. Clarke also noted that even in advanced BPH transient remissions in clinical symptoms of the disease occurred in almost 60% of patients for approximately one year. Castro et al.[57], in a double-blind study, found improvement in frequency and nocturia in approximately 70% of placebo-treated patients over six months.

(2) Objective measurements are preferred for assessing therapy in patients with BPH treated with drugs.

The hallmark of BPH is increased urethral resistance secondary to a decrease in effective cross-sectional area of the urethra. Increased urethral resistance can be derived mathematically from measurement of maximal urinary flow rate and maximal intravesical pressure, and separates patients with BPH from normals quite readily. Castro and Griffiths[57] showed a correlation coefficient between maximal urine flow rates and urethral cross-sectional areas to be $r = 0.96$. Furthermore, Castro et al. found in a double-blind study that maximal urine flow rate remained unchanged in placebo-treated patients.

Residual urine obtained by catheter measurements also shows a reliable objective correlation with urethral resistance. Castro has reported residual urine measurements by three different techniques in placebo-treated patients as part of a double-blind assessment for the effects of aldactone in BPH. He states that radiographic measurements are unsuitable for assessments of residual urine. He points out that in a group of placebo-treated patients followed over six months, there was significant decrease in planimetrically measured residual urine in both the intravenous pyelogram and retrograde cystogram, although the residual urine, measured by catheterization, remained constant. Data reported by Clarke[2], and Wolfe and Madsen[58] also indicates that residual urine measured by catheter over six or more months is not likely to show spontaneous sustained decreases of any significance. Ability to void, in patients with established chronic retention and indwelling catheters, is a valid objective criterion if controls for the effect of catheter drainage itself are included.

(3) Histological change by open biopsy is an objective technique if the examination is quantified, as exemplified in the report of Huggins and Stevens[11]. Biopsies are not suitable, since the needle itself, may produce artifacts and significant variation in the tissue. Other so-called objective criteria are not reliable, but have been employed as criteria in drug studies. These include:

a. Rectal examination. Castro et al.[57], have shown that there is no correlation between rectal size and urethral resistance.

b. Length of prostatic urethra. Castro et al.[59], have shown this does not correlate with urethral resistance.

c. Prostate size measurement by cytourethrogram. Zelefsky[60] has indicated that variations in studies performed in the same patient a few minutes apart show a significant standard deviation of $\pm 25\%$, and therefore are not precise enough for use as an indicator of change in prostate size.

In summary, the acceptable objective criteria suitable for the study of drug effects in BPH, when the patient is his own control, are: (1) urine flow rate changes; (2) catheterized residual urine changes; (3) ability to void, in patients with established urinary retention; and (4) quantitative histologic changes in prostates obtained from open resection.

If subjective criteria are to be used, then adequate placebo-treated controls with double-blind technique must be used, or else studies should be conducted for a minimum of three years.

DELALUTIN AND CHLORMADINONE ACETATE STUDIES

The first study of a progestational anti-androgen was done by Geller[47], who studied ten patients without controls and with some objective techniques, including residual urine and quantitative histologic changes in several of the patients. Aware of the deficiency of this initial study, Geller[61] then selected eleven patients with BPH for study, ten of whom had established urinary retention as indicated by inability to void on at least two trials conducted ten or more days apart. One of the eleven patients had established increased residual urine of 200 ml but was able to void spontaneously prior to the study. Of the ten patients in retention, seven had indwelling Foley catheters and three had cystotomy tubes. To control the effect of the catheter or tube as therapy, a control series of ten patients with indwelling Foley catheters or cystotomy tubes was studied over a three-month period, with repeated trials of voiding. Among the ten patients in retention treated for at least four months, five out of the seven on Delalutin and two out of the three on Chlormadinone acetate voided spontaneously, with residual urines of less than 50 ml by five months following treatment (Table 2.3). Residual urine in the eleventh patient decreased from 200 ml to a negligible amount in four months. There were three treatment failures, two on Delalutin and one on Chlormadinone acetate. In patient number 2 (Table 2.3) initial improvement on Delalutin was followed by retention three months after the drug was discontinued.

In the control group of ten patients with BPH who were in urinary retention, only two voided spontaneously after three months of catheter or cystotomy tube drainage alone. Comparison of the ability to void in the control and treated groups indicated a statistically significant difference between them, using a Chi-square test (Table 2.4). A second control group used for that same study was taken from the paper of Clarke[2] which indicated the rarity of spontaneous decrease in residual urine to less than 50 ml once an elevated residual urine was established. Since then, both Wolfe and Madsen[58], and Castro[59], have reported that untreated controls with BPH, with established increased residual urine, had no change in this variable over a six-month follow-up period.

Table 2.3 EFFECT OF PROGESTATIONAL AGENTS ON ABILITY TO VOID AND RESIDUAL URINE IN PATIENTS WITH BPH DURING AND FOLLOWING THERAPY

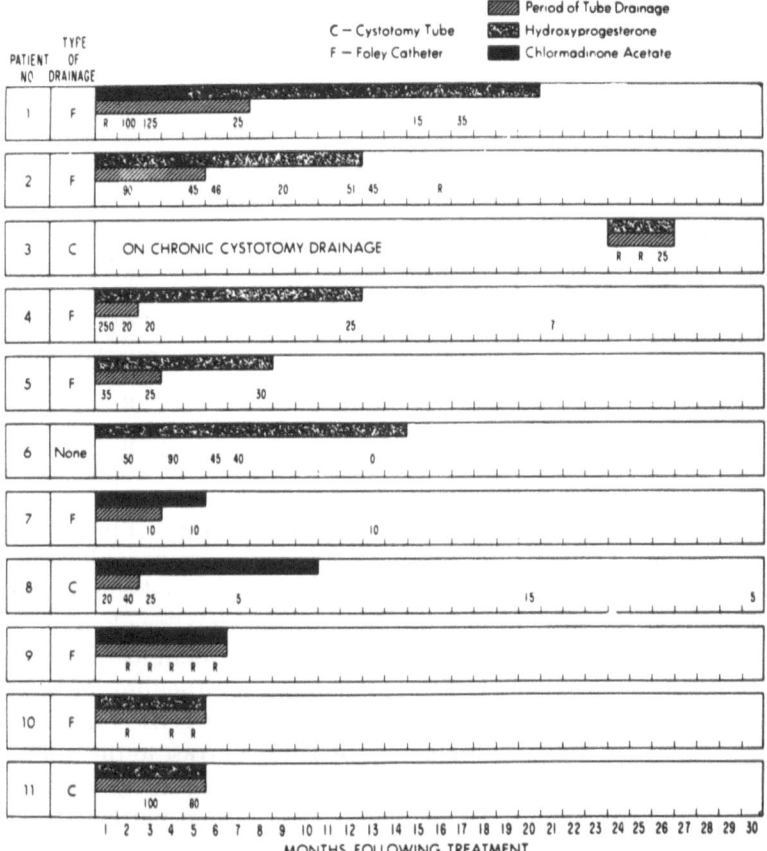

This table presents data from 11 individual patients with BPH treated with either hydroxyprogesterone or chlormadinone acetate. The relationship of drug therapy to cystotomy tube or Foley catheter drainage and to residual urine and ability to void during and following the tube drainage is depicted for each patient. The numbers shown at the bottom of each patient bar refer to the residual urine at that particular time. "R" indicates urinary retention.

Other objective criteria in Geller's studies were histologic studies of openly resected prostates which showed that the epithelial cells in treated specimens tended to be more cuboidal in many areas in lieu of the tall columnar cells reported by

Table 2.4 RESIDUAL URINE FOLLOWING CATHETER DRAINAGE IN
PATIENTS WITH URINARY RETENTION

Patient	Before catheter drainage	2 Months after catheter drainage
1 (F)	R	R
2 (F)	R	R
3 (F)	R	R
4 (F)	R	30 ml
5 (F)	R	R
6 (F)	R	R
7 (F)	R	80 ml
8 (C)	R	10 ml
9 (C)	R	R
10 (C)	R	R

F indicates Foley catheter; C, cystotomy tube; R, retention.

others. In sections from hydroxyprogesterone-treated patients,
there seemed to be fewer nodules in the same comparable area
of the prostate. In general, nodules were smaller and contained
fewer and less distended acini. In addition, smaller glandular
acini were seen. Another difference was the evident loss or only
minimal papillation of lining glandular epithelium in the
treated patients, even in areas of tall columnar cells. The cells
showed mid-zonal positioning of nuclei in contrast to the more
basal position of the untreated group. The basal cells were a
bit more prominent in the section from a treated patient.

In the treated group, the stroma was composed mostly of
rather mature smooth muscle cells. No evident fibrotic changes
were demonstrable with certainty (Figure 2.3).

One of the most interesting findings of Geller's study with
Delalutin was the prolonged remission in four out of five
patients during an average follow-up of thirteen months after
discontinuation of the drug. This suggests that the factors,
hormonal or otherwise, which produce BPH over probably
many years may not recur following successful therapy. Effective therapy, therefore, may be used intermittently and not
necessarily be required for life. In the Delalutin studies,

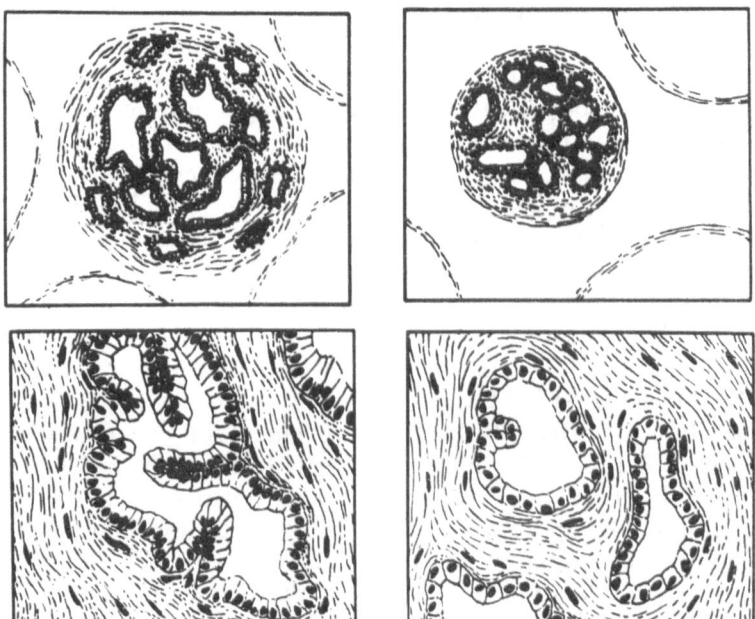

Figure 2.3   Composite diagram of histologic changes in prostate during progestational hormone therapy

Top. In the treated group (right) smaller nodular areas and smaller glandular acini are noted than in those of the untreated group (left)

Bottom. Glandular epithelium in untreated group (left) shows tall columnar epithelial cells with basal nuclei and abundant papillary projections. Treated group (right) shows cuboidal to columnar epithelial cells with basal to midzonal nuclei, less and inconspicuous papillation

endocrine evaluation indicated a significant decrease in plasma testosterone levels without significant changes in pituitary gonadotropins or adrenal cortical steroids, pointing to a direct inhibitory effect of the drug of testosterone synthesis.

In two subsequent published studies using Delalutin, one by Weinberg[62] and one by Jacobs et al.[63], negative results were reported. In Weinberg's study of fifteen patients, patients received 2.5 g/week rather than 3 g, as used by Geller. Five of Weinberg's patients had either bladder stones or urethral strictures, and therefore were not examples of BPH. In the remaining ten patients, three received therapy for one month or less. No objective criteria were used, and no controls were employed. This study must be considered inadequate. Jacobs studied the effect of Delalutin in twenty patients for three months. Although the residual urine was measured, individual values related to duration of therapy are not given, and the total number of patients studied for changes in residual urine is not noted in the article. In summary, the Geller study, while small in numbers, strongly suggests the effectiveness of Delalutin for BPH, as based upon several of the established and acceptable objective criteria. Lack of adequate number of patients, lack of controls for clinical parameters, and incomplete studies of objective factors such as urine flow rate, make the study inconclusive.

19-NOR-DELALUTIN

Crooks[64] reported objective improvement in five of seven patients in maximal urinary flow treated with 19-Nor-Delalutin. Subjective improvement was also noted over a three-month follow-up, but the lack of controls invalidates the usefulness of this part of the study. Vahlensieck et al.[65], treated five inoperable BPH patients with 300 mg per week of 19-Nor-Delalutin for two to four months. All five had elevated residual urines which decreased significantly. Catheterized residual urine values ranged from 150–1200 ml before therapy, and from 0–200 ml after therapy. Three of the five patients had values less than 100 ml post therapy. Other favorable effects of the drug were noted such as decreased rectal size and improved voiding, but these criteria were either non-objective or not controlled. Two of the five patients were catheterized, and the effects of the catheter itself were not controlled in the study.

A larger study of the effect of 19-Nor-Delalutin on BPH was done by Nuri et al.[66], who reported good subjective results in 41 patients. No controls were included, and therefore the subjective improvement following 19-Nor-Delalutin is not interpretable. One objective criterion used, however, was residual urine. Unfortunately, three of the patients with initially elevated residual urine that decreased to less than 50 ml after therapy were catheterized for several weeks at the start of treatment. No controls for the effect of the catheter were included, therefore, the change in residual urine as a valid objective parameter must be questioned in these few patients. Nevertheless, in patients with greater than 50 ml residual urine who were not catheterized, 86% showed a decrease in residual urine. Certainly part of this study must be considered as adequately objective and positive for a drug effect.

CYPROTERONE ACETATE AND NORLUTIN

Two authors have reported the effects of cyproterone acetate (Cyp A) in patients with BPH. Scott and Wade[49] administered 50 mg per day of Cyp A to thirteen patients with BPH. They measured residual urine and urine flow rates and reported that both of these objectives criteria improved in the majority of patients. Uncontrolled subjective parameters were also said to improve during the course of study. Vahlensieck[65] has also reported favorable effects of Cyp A in patients with BPH. He used, as acceptable objective criteria, the residual urine in a group of twelve patients treated for an average of three months with Cyp A, 100 mg per day. These favorable reports (along with the clinical experience with Cyp A in carcinoma of the prostate, where it appears to be effective and without significant side effects) indicate that this drug is a most promising agent for the management of BPH.

Wolfe and Madsen[58] studied the effect of Norlutin, 5 mg per day, in a well controlled, but not double-blind study over six months, involving 18 treated patients and 20 controls. They measured residual urine and urine flow rates, as well as subjective symptoms. These authors were unable to find any effect of the test drug on objective signs or subjective symptoms of BPH. This negative study has been questioned, both because of the small dose of drug employed as well as the fact that the drug metabolizes into an estrogen as measured in urine.

MEGESTROL ACETATE

Lebech and Nordentoft[67] studied the effect of megestrol acetate in fifteen randomly selected patients with BPH who were followed over a ten-month period. Their overall results indicated a favorable drug effect. Since they did not include controls or double-blind technique, the part of their study which included non-objective measurements such as cystoscopy, intravenous urography and cystourethrography cannot be considered significant findings. However, they did include measurements of residual urine and urine flow rates, both of which are valid objective criteria. In their study, residual urine averaged 200 ml prior to therapy; six months later this had decreased significantly to 30 ml. Similarly, urine flow rates showed a significant increase from 3 ml per sec to 7 ml per sec in six months.

MEDROGESTONE
Perhaps the most carefully done study to date of the effects of progestational anti-androgens in patients with BPH was published by Rangno et al.[68], who studied medrogestone in 24 patients over a twelve-month period. Criteria studied included frequency, nocturia, hesitancy, intermittency, force and size of stream, prostate size, intravenous pyelogram, cystogram, cystoscopy and radioactive residual urine. Since they used controls and double-blind technique for an adequate period of observation, their findings of a significant favorable effect of the test drug, both on clinical and objective parameters, must be considered the most convincing evidence to date.

A summary of the clinical results obtained with these eight different anti-androgens in a total of thirteen studies is shown in Table 2.2.

In addition to the progestational anti-androgens, Aldactone has also been used as a clinical therapeutic agent in patients with BPH. Fingerhut and Veenema[69] suggested that Aldactone was useful in 60–65% of patients with BPH. However, Castro and Griffiths[57], in a double-blind, controlled, clinical study, found that spironolactone was not better than a placebo for short-term treatment for BPH over a six-month period.

SUMMARY
Of ten studies in the literature in which acceptable objective criteria are used, nine report favorable effects of progestational anti-androgens in BPH (Table 2.2). One negative study of Wolfe and Madsen[58] used Norlutin in a low dosage of 5 mg per day; Norlutin is also metabolized to estrogen.

During the course of these studies, the importance of a new endocrine dimension has been appreciated; namely, the intracellular endocrine compartment. Such a compartment may contain hormones which differ both qualitatively and quantitatively from the extracellular fluid compartment. Perhaps an adequate explanation for the development of BPH will become available when studies of intracellular hormone levels are completed. Thus, far, an abnormality in intracellular DHT, which has not been confirmed, stands out as an important clue to the possible pathogenesis of BPH. The presence of functioning testicular tissue is an incontestable prerequisite for the development of BPH. Since the testis produces at least two hormones, estrogen and androgen, the concept that a disturbance of estrogen and androgen levels or their ratio may result in BPH seems reasonable. Indeed, current accurate steroid assay techniques indicate a decrease in the androgen:estrogen ratio, as measured by urine metabolites, in patients with BPH.

But what about the intracellular levels of these hormones, especially since enzymes for converting testosterone to DHT and other reduced metabolites exist within the prostate? The conversion of testosterone to estrogen, and estrogen into 2-hydroxylated and 2-methylated compounds within the prostate has been reported. The ambisexual embryologic origin of the prostate appears well established and constitutes strong evidence to justify the importance of studying estrogen metabolism, both in the normal development of the prostate and particularly in the development of BPH.

It seems likely that progestational anti-androgens are clinically effective in patients with BPH. One of these drugs, cyproterone acetate, can produce virtual medical castration as regards circulating and excreted sex steroids. Data thus far indicates that the intracellular androgen biochemical pathway is blocked by cyproterone acetate. No data concerning effects of this drug on intracellular estrogen have been reported, and conclusive evidence for the effect of the usefulness of drug therapy will depend upon larger and well-controlled clinical studies. Techniques are now available that should allow a comparison of intracellular hormone levels in patients with BPH to controls. Once established, such studies may uncover a biochemical abnormality in prostates of patients with BPH. This could then lead to the establishment of a study of a suitable drug to correct the biochemical abnormality. An adequate double-blind study would ultimately be required to establish the efficacy of medical therapy for BPH.

Since carcinoma of the prostate is common and may co-exist in the same age groups as BPH, it is important to consider the effect of the drug to be used on a possible latent carcinoma of the prostate. Cyproterone acetate has already been reported by Geller[70] to have beneficial effects in carcinoma of the prostate.

Finally, the side effects of many drugs to be studied must be considered, since long-term therapy involving many patients is anticipated. At least one of these drugs, cyproterone acetate, decreases libido. It does not produce thromboembolic complications or uniform changes in glucose tolerance; gynecomastia occurs rarely, if at all. There are rare reports of transaminase changes in patients treated with cyproterone acetate; neither weight loss nor other catabolic effects have been noted. It is of interest that progestational agents have now been employed successfully to treat Type V hyper-lipidemias.

These drugs, progestational anti-androgens, therefore constitute a very hopeful prototype for the ultimate medical management of benign prostatic hypertrophy.

REFERENCES

1. Flocks, R. H. (1964). Benign prostatic hypertrophy: its diagnosis and management. *Med. Times*, *92*, 519
2. Clarke, Roscoe (1937). The prostate and the endocrines: a control series. *Brit. J. Urol.*, *9*, 254
3. Chang, H. L. and Char, G. Y. (1936). Benign hypertrophy of the prostate. *Chinese Med. J.*, *50*, 1707
4. D'Aunoy, R., Schenken, J. R. and Burns, E. L. (1939). The relative incidence of hyperplasia of the prostate in the white and colored races in Louisiana. *Southern Med. J.*, *32*, 47
5. Derbes, V. de P., Leche, S. M. and Hooker, C. W. (1937). The incidence of benign prostatic hypertrophy among the whites and negroes in New Orleans. *J. Urol.*, *38*, 383
6. Moore, R. A. (1944). Benign hypertrophy and carcinoma of the prostate. Occurrence and experimental production in animals. *Surgery*, *16*, 152
7. Hunter, John (1786). 'Observations on the glands situated between the rectum and the bladder, called vesiculae seminales'. In *Collected Works*, vol. 4, p. 31, edited by J. F. Palmer, London

8. Zuckerman, S. (1936). The endocrine control of the prostate. *Proc. Roy. Soc. Med.*, *29*, 1557

9. White, J. W. (1895). The results of double castration in hypertrophy of the prostate. *Ann. Surg.*, *22*, 1

10. Cabot, A. T. (1896). The question of castration for enlarged prostate. *Ann. Surg.*, *24*, 265

11. Huggins, C. and Stevens, R. A. (1940). The effect of castration of benign hypertrophy of the prostate in man. *J. Urol.*, *43*, 705

12. Callow, R. K. and Deanesly, R. (1935). Effect of androsterone and of male hormone concentrates on accessory reproductive organs of castrated rats, mice, and guinea pigs. *Biochem. J.*, *29*, 1424

13. Lacassagne, A. (1933). Metaplasie Epidermoide de la prostate provoquee chez la souris par des injections repetees des fortes doses de Folliculine. *C.R. Soc. Biol. (Paris)*, *113*, 590

14. de Jongh, S. E. (1933). Geschlechtshormone and Schleimhautabstossung im mannilichen Genitalapparat (Demonstration). *Acta Brev. Neerl.*, *3*, 112

15. Korenchevsky, V. and Dennison, M. (1934). Effect of oestrone on normal and castrated male rats. *Biochem. J.*, *28*, 1474

16. Burrows, H. and Kennaway, N. M. (1934). On some effects produced by applying oestin to the skin of mice. *Amer. J. Cancer*, *20*, 48

17. Van Cappellen, D. (1936). The treatment of benign hypertrophy with preparations of the male sex hormone. *Brit. J. Urol.*, *8*, 8

18. Morell, T. (1934). Therapeutische Ergahrungen mit einum neuen Volleitrakt aus Mannlichen Keimdrusen (Androstina). *Deutsch Med. Wschr.*, *60*, 1516

19. Schmitz, G. (1937). Erfahrungen mit dem neuen synthetischen testeshormono-praparat Perandren. *Deutsch Med. Wschr.*, *63*, 230

20. Emmens, C. W. and Parkes, A. S. (1938). Oestrogens of testis and of adrenal in relation to treatment of enlarged prostate with testosterone propionate. *J. Path. Bact.*, *47*, 279

21. Strohm, J. G., Edelson, Z. C. and Merryman, G. H. (1938). The clinical use of testosterone in the treatment of benign prostatic hypertrophy. *Urol. and Cutan. Rev.*, *42*, 510

22. Walther, H. W. E. and Willoughby, R. M. (1938). Hormonal treatment of benign prostate hyperplasia. *J. Urol.*, *40*, 135

23. Moore, R. A. and McLellan, A. M. (1938). A histological study of the effect of the sex hormones on the human prostate. *J. Urol.*, *40*, 641

24. Heckel, N. J. (1940). The influence of testosterone-propionate upon benign prostatic hypertrophy and spermatogenesis: A clinical and pathological study in the human. *J. Urol.*, *43*, 286

25. Lower, W. E., Engel, W. J. and McCullagh, D. R. (1935). A summary of the experimental research on the control of benign prostatic hypertrophy and a preliminary clinical report. *J. Urol.*, *34*, 670

26. McCullagh, D. R. and Walsh, E. L. (1935). Experimental hypertrophy and atrophy of the prostate gland. *Endocrinology*, *19*, 216

27. Chwalla, R. (1954). Prostatic disease. *J. Amer. Med. Ass.*, *155*, 852

28. Stumpf, H. H. and Wilens, S. L. (1953). Inhibiting effects of portal cirrhosis of the liver on prostatic enlargement. *Arch. Intern. Med. (Chicago)*, *91*, 304

29. Robson, M. C. (1964). The incidence of benign prostatic hyperplasia and prostatic carcinoma in cirrhosis of the liver. *J. Urol.*, *92*, 307

30. Kahle, J. J. and Maltry, E. (1940). Treatment of hyperplasia of the prostate with diethylstilbestrol and diethylstilbestrol dipropionate: a preliminary report. *New Orleans Med. Surg. J.*, *93*, 121

31. Cook, E. N. (1963). Diagnosis and treatment of benign prostatic hyperplasia. *Postgrad. Med.*, *33*, 446

32. Vernon, S. (1958). Nocturia in the elderly male. *J. Amer. Geriat. Soc.*, *6*, 411

33. Roberts, H. J. (1966). Estrogenic management of benign prostatism, including early and poor-risk cases: 7-year experience. *J. Amer. Geriat. Soc.*, *14*, 657

34. Heckel, N. J. (1944). Evaluation of sex hormones in the treatment of benign prostatic hypertrophy, carcinoma of the prostate and other diseases of the genito-urinary system. *J. Clin. Endocr.*, *4*, 166

35. Moszkowicz, L. (1935). Die Prostata der Zwetter und die Systematic des Zwetter-tums. *Virchow Arch. Path. Anat.*, *295*, 211

36. Wilkins, Lawson (1948). A feminizing adrenal tumor causing gynecomastia in a boy of five years contrasted with a virilizing tumor in a five-year-old girl. *J. Clin. Endocr.*, *8*, 111

37. Bauer, K. (1951). Combined treatment of prostatic hypertrophy with both sex hormones or gonad extracts. *Deutsch Med. Wschr.*, *76*, 1456

38. Kaufman, J. J. and Goodwin, W. E. (1959). Hormonal management of the benign obstructing prostate: Use of combined androgen-estrogen therapy. *J. Urol.*, *81*, 165

39. Kaufmann, J. (1968). Untersuchungen zur kausalen Genese der Prostatehyper-trophie. II. Teil. *Z. Urol.*, *4*, 229

40. Segal, S. J. and Nelson, W. O. (1958). Recent progress in the endocrinology of reproduction. Proceeding of the Conference held in Syracuse, New York, June 9–12, 1958. Edited by Charles W. Lloyd, New York: Academic Press

41. Nagai, N. and Longcope, C. (1971). Estradiol-17β and estrone: Studies on their binding to rabbit uterine cytosol and the concentration in plasma. *Steroids*, *17*, 631

42. Geller, J., Baron, A. and Kleinman, S. (1970). Pituitary luteinizing hormone reserve in elderly men with prostatic disease. *J. Endocr.*, *48*, 289

43. Grayhack, J. T., Bunce, P. L., Kearns, J. W. and Scott, W. W. (1955). Influence of the pituitary on prostatic response to androgen in the rat. *Bull. Johns Hopkins Hosp.*, *96*, 154

44. Asano, M. (1965). Basic experimental studies of the pituitary prolactin-prostate interrelationships. *J. Urol.*, *93*, 97

45. Fang, S. and Liao, S. (1971). Androgen receptors: Steroid- and tissue-specific retention of a 17β-hydroxy-5α-androstan-3-one-protein complex by the cell nuclei of ventral prostate. *J. Biol. Chem.*, *246*, 16

46. Siiteri, P. K. and Wilson, J. D. (1970). Dihydrotestosterone in prostatic hyper-trophy. I. The formation and content of dihydrotestosterone in the hypertrophic prostate of man. *J. Clin. Invest.*, *49*, 1737

47. Geller, J., Bork, R., Roberts, T., Newman, H., Lin, A. and Silva, R. (1965). Treatment of benign prostatic hypertrophy with hydroxyprogesterone caproate. *J. Amer. Med. Ass.*, *193*, 121

48. Geller, J., Fruchtman, B., Meyer, C. and Newman, H. (1967). Effect of pro-gestational agents on gonadal and adrenal cortical function in patients with

benign prostatic hypertrophy and carcinoma of the prostate. *J. Clin. Endocr.*, *27*, 556

49. Scott, W. W. and Wade, J. C. (1969). Medical treatment of benign nodular prostatic hyperplasia with cyproterone acetate. *J. Urol.*, *101*, 81

50. Fishman, J. and Geller, J. (1970). Effect of the anti-androgen cyproterone acetate on estradiol production and metabolism in man. *Steroids*, *16*, 351

51. Geller, J. (1972). Unpublished data

52. Hansson, V. and Tveter, K. J. (1971). Effect of anti-androgens on the uptake and binding of androgen by human benign nodular prostatic hyperplasia in vitro. *Acta Endocrinol. (Kbh)*, *68*, 69

53. Geller, J., van Damme, O., Garabieta, G., Loh, A., Rettura, J. and Seifter, E. (1969). Effect of cyproterone acetate on ^{3}H-testosterone uptake and anzyme synthesis by the ventral prostate of the rat. *Endocrinology*, *84*, 1330

54. Farnsworth, W. E. (1966). Metabolism of 19-nortestosterone by human prostate. *Steroids*, *8*, 826

55. Acevedo, H. F. and Goldzieher, J. W. (1965). The metabolism of [14C] estrone by hypertrophic and carcinomatous human prostate tissue. *Biochim. Biophys. Acta.*, *97*, 571

56. Unhjem, O. and Tveter, K. J. (1969). Localization of an androgen binding substance from the rat ventral prostate. *Acta Endocrinol. (Kbh)*, *60*, 571

57. Castro, J. E. and Griffiths, H. L. J. (1972). The assessment of patients with benign prostatic hypertrophy. *J. Roy. Coll. Surg. Edinburgh*, *17*, 190

58. Wolf, H. and Madsen, P. O. (1968). Treatment of benign prostatic hypertrophy with progestational agents: A preliminary report. *J. Urol.*, *99*, 780

59. Castro, J. E., Griffiths, H. J. L. and Shackman, R. (1969). Significance of signs and symptoms in benign prostatic hypertrophy. *Brit. Med. J.*, *2*, 598

60. Zelefsky, M. (1968). Precision of anatomic mensuration from roentgenograms: A cystourethrographic study. *Amer. J. Roentgen*, *104*, 372

61. Geller, J., Angrist, A., Nakao, K. and Newman, H. (1969). Therapy with progestational agents in advanced benign prostatic hypertrophy. *J. Amer. Med. Ass.*, *210*, 1421

62. Weinberg, S. R. (1968). Refractoriness of prostatism to hydroxyprogesterone capronate (Delalutin) therapy. *J. Urol.*, *100*, 57

63. Jacobs, D., Harper, J. M. and Politano, V. A. (1967). Evaluation of hydroxyprogesterone caproate in the treatment of benign prostatic hyperplasia. *Southern Med. J.*, *60*, 1174

64. Crooks, J. (1968). Unpublished data

65. Vahlensieck, W. and St. Godde (1968). Behandlung der Prostatahypertrophie mit Gestagenen. *Munchen Med. Wschr.*, *110*, 1573

66. Nuri, M. and Hochberg, K. (1970). Behandlung der Prostata-Hypertrophie mid Depostat. *Munchen Med. Wschr.*, *112*, 1057

67. Lebech, P. E. and Nordentoft, E. L. (1967). A study of endocrine function in the treatment of benign prostatic hypertrophy with Megestrol Acetate. *Acta Obstet. Gynaecol. Scand.*, *46*, (Suppl. 9), 25

68. Rangno, R. E., McLeod, P. J., Ruedy, J. and Ogilvie, R. I. (1971). Treatment of benign prostatic hypertrophy with medrogestone. *Clin. Pharmacol. Therap.*, *12*, 658

69. Fingerhut, B. and Veenema, R. J. (1967). The effect of bilateral adrenalectomy on induced benign prostatic hyperplasia in mice. *J. Urol.*, *97*, 508

70. Geller, J., Vazakas, G., Fruchtman, B., Newman, H., Nakao, K. and Loh, A. (1968). The effect of cyproterone acetate on advanced carcinoma of the prostate. *Surg. Gynecol. Obstet.*, *127*, 748

71. Isurugi, K. (1967). Plasma testosterone production rates in patients with prostatic cancer and benign prostatic hypertrophy. *J. Urol.*, *97*, 903

72. Rivarola, M. A., Saez, J. M., Meyer, W. J., Jenkins, M. E. and Migeon, C. J. (1966). Metabolic clearance rate and blood production rate of testosterone and androst-4-ene-3,17-dione under basal conditions, ACTH and HCG stimulation: Comparison with urinary production rate of testosterone. *J. Clin. Endocrinol.*, *26*, 1208

73. Hudson, B., Coghlan, J. P. and Dulmanis, A. (1967). *Ciba Foundation Colloquia on Endocrinology*, Vol. XVI, by G. Wolstenholme and M. O'Connor, editors. Boston: Little, Brown and Company

74. Ismail, A. A. and Harkness, R. A. (1967). Urinary testosterone excretion in men in normal and pathological conditions. *Acta Endocrinol. (Kbh)*, *56*, 469

75. Morer-Fargas, R. and Nowakowski, H. (1965). Die testosteronausscheidung im ham bei Mannlichen Individuen. *Acta Endocrinol. (Kbh)*, *49*, 443

76. Kent, J. R. and Acone, A. B. (1966). *Excerpta Medica Foundation*, Amsterdam, International Congress Series No. 101, p. 31

3

Surgery of benign prostatic hypertrophy

J. P. Mitchell

Historical landmarks in prostatectomy

Although the anatomy of the prostate gland is thought to have
been appreciated by the ancient Chinese and early Egyptian
writers and descriptions by Susruta and Galen are thought to
refer to the prostate gland, it is impossible to determine whether
they appreciated the significant difference between the prostate, the seminal vesicles and the ampullae of the vasa. The
distinction made by Bartholinus[1] was limited to the term
'little stones' for the lobes of the prostate, to differentiate them
from the 'true stones'.

Similarly, although factors causing obstruction to the
urinary flow were described by numerous writers up to and
including the middle ages, it is again impossible to determine
whether the carnosities and caruncles to which they refer
were, in fact, descriptions of hypertrophy of the bladder neck
and prostate or stricture of the urethra.

Catheters fit to wear afunder, or tear Caruncles.

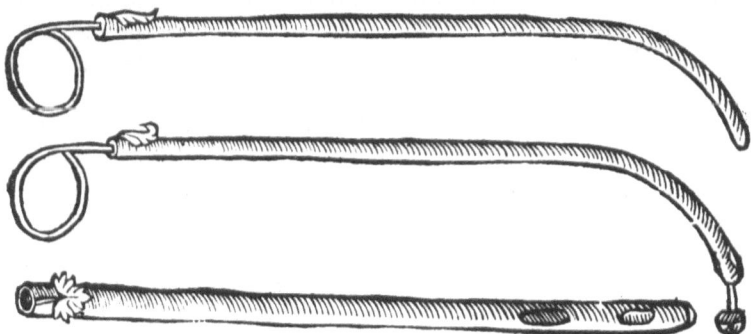

Figure 3.1 A leaden catheter with rough button for breaking and tearing of caruncles
from Ambroise Paré's Introduction to Chirurgery 1691

Although Ambroise Paré[2] is credited with the earliest accurate description of symptoms of prostatism, even he makes no distinction between the obstruction from stricture of the urethra, and the obstruction due to an enlargement of the prostate and, again, both conditions are described under the same heading of 'carnosities'. He has, in fact, often been quoted as "passing a sound to which is attached a fin for cutting the neck of the bladder", but I have been quite unable to confirm this in any of his literature, though Figure 3.1 shows his "leaden catheter having a rough button at the end, like a round file". This he "thrust up and down the urethra as long and as often" as he thought fit for the "breaking and tearing of the caruncles".

Yet another difficulty arises in deciding whether historical writers were in fact aware of the difference between adenomatous enlargement of the prostate and neoplasm of the bladder. As late as the 18th Century Chopart[3] and Desault[4] described 'fungus excrescences' which, according to them "may occur in any part of the bladder, even the fundus of the viscus, but at the same time they may arise near the bladder neck as a swelling of the uvula of the bladder which causes retention of urine".

It was, in fact, John Hunter[5] who first in 1788 described an anatomical analysis of the prostate gland into its lateral lobes and middle lobe, hyperplasia of which could affect the bladder musculature and also cause dilatation of the upper urinary tract. He described how the sides of the urethral canal are compressed together producing obstruction to the passage of urine. He also suggested that the middle lobe swells forward into the bladder acting like a valve to the mouth of the urethra. He also appreciated how the enlargement of the middle lobe causes the urethra to turn or bend forward, forming an obstruction to the passage of the catheter. It is an interesting quirk of history that his brother-in-law, Everard Home[6], should have been credited with the description of the subtrigonal enlargement of the prostate, even though the main concentration of his thesis is in fact on the middle lobe described previously and accurately by John Hunter.

The developments of surgery to the prostate and bladder neck during the 19th Century are well known to all urologists from the work of Guthrie, Mercier and Civiale[7-11], culminating at the end of the century in the work of surgeons such as Henry Thompson, Reginald Harrison, Gouley, Goodfellow and McGill[12-16]. At the turn of the century the controversy raged over the merits of complete or incomplete removal of the prostate, Freyer[17] making his much disputed claim to priority in the field of complete prostatectomy. A full review of the history of bladder neck and prostatic surgery would occupy more than the time and space permitted here.

Throughout the history of prostatectomy the major problem dogging all attempts at enucleation or resection were hemorrhages and infection, the latter being in large measure an aggravating factor of the hemorrhage. Various devices from hemostatic packs to Pilcher's bags were designed to exert compression within the cavity from which the prostate had been enucleated. Blood clot and subsequent pus formation were evacuated and drained via suprapubic tubes of gargantuan size, and even some of us still in practice today can remember the routine use of the Hamilton Irving box and vast numbers of offensive moss packs to absorb and drain the infected urine from the inevitable suprapubic fistula.

A variety of hemostatic sutures were described. Thomson-Walker[18], conscious of the location of the major arteries, inserted a single stitch at 4 o'clock and 8 o'clock passing through the prostatic cavity into the bladder.

Although Harris[19] of Sydney, Australia, had been credited with the first attempt to perform a prostatectomy as a one stage operation, closing the bladder completely, he was in fact preceded in this by a number of surgeons: Kümmel[20] and Duval[21] for example, but for all these other writers this was only an occasional procedure if they felt that the bleeding was not excessive immediately after enucleation. Harris's great contribution to surgery of the prostate was that he was one of the first to make a routine surgical attempt at hemostasis, apart from the use of packs, compression bags and hemostatic tampons. His objective was to close the prostatic cavity by obliterating it with two series of sutures: the first of these he called retrigonization which, in effect, was an attempt to draw the distal part of the trigone down towards the upper end of the residual urethra, so closing off the posterior part of the prostatic cavity. His next stitch was an anterior transverse suture obliterating the anterior part of the prostatic cavity and closing it onto the catheter. In the opinion of many urologists, this was the greatest advance in the surgical technique of prostatectomy, and the three important surgical principles were achieved, namely: hemostasis, reconstruction of the operation site, and primary closure of the bladder and wound.

In 1945 Wilson Hey[22] of Manchester made his great plea for asepsis and antisepsis in prostatic surgery, thus reducing considerably the amount of post-operative bleeding and leaking fistulae. In fact, to watch Wilson Hey carry out his operation, one could not help feeling that the most important feature of his surgery was the extensive hemostasis carried out with diathermy around the neck of the bladder and even down into the prostatic cavity itself. He would spend as long as three-quarters of an hour after enucleation dealing meticulously with every bleeding point he could see, and only when he considered the field was dry would he close the bladder. In the same year Terence Millin[23] made history in prostatic surgery by his description of the retropubic approach to the prostate. Here again, hemostasis was his chief contribution in that, by incising transversely the anterior wall of the capsule of the prostate, he was dividing and controlling some of the major bleeding vessels. In addition, he provided a much freer and clearer exposure of the bladder neck and prostatic cavity, so that the major vessels bleeding from 4 o'clock and 8 o'clock could be coagulated or tied accurately and vessels in the depths of the prostatic cavity could be exposed and either coagulated or oversewn. Four years later, Hryntschak[24] of Vienna described his modification of Harris's operation in which he popularized the excision of the posterior part of the bladder neck. Otherwise, in principle, his operation was identical to that of Harris. In fact, even the resection of the posterior part of the bladder neck had been described previously by both Wilson Hey and Terence Millin.

All of these earlier surgeons had been describing techniques which have contributed to the degree of hemostasis possible at prostatectomy today. Hemostasis is still the basic technical requirement of this operation and even now, with modern technology, the most skilled urologist will admit that

occasionally he runs into alarming hemorrhage after enucleation or transurethral resection of the prostate. It requires a
cool head and methodical procedure to deal with heavy
venous bleeding from the multiple venous plexi around and
within the prostatic cavity. As with surgery in any other field,
uncontrolled hemorrhage can precipitate the anxious surgeon
into rash manoeuvres which he knows are liable to cause
serious and permanent damage either to the sphincter mechanism at the lower end of the prostate or, worse still, to the
integrity of the prostatic capsule and the wall of the rectum
immediately behind. These problems are just as likely to occur
at open surgery as at transurethral resection.

The prime objective in all forms of prostatic surgery,
therefore, should be an operation which achieves maximum
hemostasis.

Indications for prostatectomy (Mitchell[25])

Broadly speaking, there are two indications for prostatectomy.
The first is some definite evidence of back pressure either on
the upper urinary tract producing hydronephrosis, or on the
lower urinary tract resulting in acute or chronic retention,
trabeculation of the bladder wall, or merely a very large
residual urine, which in fact is the early stage of chronic
retention. The second indication for prostatectomy is the inconvenience that the enlarged gland causes to the patient.
Occasionally a patient with benign prostatic hypertrophy will
present with hematuria. This may occur only once or twice, or
it may persist for several days. It is, of course, essential to
exclude any other cause for the hematuria by intravenous
pyelography and by cystoscopy, but hematuria from an enlarged prostate is not *per se* an indication for prostatectomy and
many of the patients will never have another bleed, or may go
many months or years before any further urinary symptoms
develop.

In those patients with symptoms of prostatism without
any clinical or radiological evidence of back pressure on the
bladder or upper urinary tract, assessment of the inconvenience
that the enlarged prostate is causing to the patient often
presents some difficulty. One patient will maintain that his

sleep is disturbed, and his broken nights are causing him distress when he only has to get up twice during the normal sleeping hours to pass water. On the other hand, some men will accept the fact that they have to wake up four or five times to pass water, but because they are able to get to sleep again immediately, they do not feel that this is sufficient to justify a major operation. Diurnal frequency can also be very variable in the inconvenience it causes to the patient. Here, however, it is usually a question of social or professional duties. The old gentleman who has to attend Board meetings or to sit on the Bench as a Magistrate may find it very embarrassing if he cannot hold his water for longer than two hours, whereas the man who has retired to a quiet life in his garden and his greenhouse probably is not aware that he passes his water every hour. Urinary incontinence is easy to assess, as this is almost invariably associated with some degree of chronic retention, the incontinence being a form of overflow. Hesitancy is a symptom which usually distresses the patient in the middle of the night when he is disturbed by the desire to pass water, and he stands for several minutes or even half-an-hour in the cold before he is able to produce a trickle of urine. Another man may be troubled by day, particularly in a public urinal when, for example, during the interval at the theatre he finds he is quite unable to produce any urine because others are present, and he has to return to his seat and endure the next act in great discomfort. Journeys by car or train can cause considerable embarrassment to the urinary flow in patients who otherwise may have little trouble with micturition. This may be due to vascular congestion or possibly to vibration transmitted to the sacrum, producing reflex spasms of the bladder neck via the nervi erigentes.

The inconvenience which prostatic symptoms cause to the patient can only be assessed by the patient himself, and it is the doctor's duty to advise the patient first as to how much relief this operation can give, and secondly on the relatively low mortality in patients who are otherwise fit.

Patients may sometimes ask, even though their symptoms at the time are minimal whether they ought to undergo the operation in view of the progressive nature of the disease and the inevitable deterioration of their physical fitness as they grow older. This form of prophylactic prostatectomy can rarely be justified in the light of modern anesthetic advances, where age alone adds comparatively little to the operative risks. Although prostatic hypertrophy is always a progressive condition, it is impossible to assess the rate at which progress will occur and no prognosis can be given on when, if ever, retention is likely to develop.

In two instances we may be forced to accept a lesser degree of symptoms as an indication for surgery. The first is that of the chronic bronchitic, who may be a very bad risk for an emergency prostatectomy in winter when his chest is at its worst, whereas the same operation for him in early summer could be a less hazardous procedure and would give him the rest of the summer months for his convalescence. The other instance where assessment is always difficult is that of the man who is going abroad for business or professional reasons or even for a prolonged holiday, perhaps to celebrate the beginning of his retirement. He is apprehensive at the thought of being rushed into hospital in a foreign country where he may not be fluent in the language and he will be far from his wife and family. Admittedly air transport has reduced this problem for the business man whose fare is paid, and who can be despatched home at short notice; but the traveller who has retired on a pension, and has probably saved for many years for this journey to foreign parts, perhaps to see one of his children who has emigrated, is faced with a serious dilemma. Here it is probably wise to accept symptoms of rather less severity and advise surgery so that he can make his journey with complete peace of mind.

Because of the age of most patients for whom prostatic surgery is contemplated, we find in the majority either some cardiac or respiratory complications, or both. A physical examination of the patient will give us little information as to whether that patient will stand anesthetic and surgery. The enquiries most helpful in assessing the physical fitness of the patient are those directed to an assessment of his mode of life during the past few months. Has he been up and about and leading a reasonably active life? Has he a garden that he looks after, or does he do the shopping for his wife? Finally, if he can get out of bed, walk round it, and get back in again without assistance, he is almost certainly fit to stand a prostatic operation.

In the severe bronchitic, post-operative control may not be achieved as quickly as in the normal patient. Repeated attacks of coughing may cause a slight loss of urine, as in the woman with stress incontinence. Usually this is only transient, but a word of warning to the patient preoperatively can save the surgeon the embarrassment of explaining in the post-operative stage. Patients readily accept an anticipated complication, whereas the post-operative development of transient incontinence, coming on without previous warning, may suggest to the patient an error in surgery.

The contra-indications to prostatic surgery are either advanced cerebral disease, or a patient bedridden because of cardiac, respiratory or locomotor failure, or a combination of these. Such bedridden patients will probably be just as well off with an indwelling catheter, and certainly much easier to manage. The post-operative results if surgery is attempted in a bedridden patient are never so successful, presumably because these patients tend to develop a sump of infected urine in the base of the bladder and pass only the clear supernatent fluid, which results in a severe basal cystitis. Even though the residual urine may be only 1 or 2 ounces, this remains in the bas fond of the bladder stagnating into thick pus.

One could almost say that no patient is too old for prostatectomy. On the other hand, the older the patient the higher is the incidence of some other complicating factor such as cerebral, cardiac, or respiratory disease. The most helpful approach in assessing an aged patient who is a prospective candidate for prostatectomy is to consider his natural expectation of life.

In the event of prostatectomy being contra-indicated, we are left with only two alternatives in a patient who already has retention, namely a permanent indwelling catheter or a permanent suprapubic cystostomy. A few patients will tolerate a suprapubic cystostomy with complete equanimity, but to the majority of patients it is irksome and even painful. Even with the development of the silastic catheter, these still need changing at 3 to 6 week intervals, depending on the speed with which the patient forms phosphatic plaques on the catheter.

Unless patients are bedridden, they will usually prefer to take the risk of surgery rather than putting up with the discomfort and inconvenience of any form of catheter. In most clinics today, few patients (less than 1%, O'Flynn[29]) are denied prostatectomy on the grounds of being unfit for surgery.

Transurethral resection of the benign prostate (Mitchell[26])

The transurethral approach for resecting the benign prostate has been an established procedure since the development of the double reflecting prism, giving a fore-oblique view (McCarthy[27]), and the design of a retractable tungsten loop, controlled by a ratchet (Stern[28]).

From that time improvements in technique have been largely due to developments in the diathermy machine, the optical system of the telescope, the smooth running of the mechanism and, finally, the introduction of hypotensive anesthesia.

The choice of approach to a benign prostate—that is to say by transurethral resection or by retropubic prostatectomy—is largely a matter of the size of the gland. A small adenoma will enucleate only with difficulty at retropubic prostatectomy, whereas the large adenoma will result in a somewhat protracted prostatectomy by the transurethral route. The comparative mortality figures (O'Flynn[29]) must be taken into account and for this reason a larger adenoma would be attempted transurethrally in a patient who was either obese or had cardio-respiratory limitation. The patient with a moderately large adenoma who is somewhat obese will probably do better with a transurethral resection taking a little longer than average, while the patient with cardio-respiratory limitations can have a staged resection if the anesthetist feels that there is any cause for anxiety. Just occasionally we have resected one lateral lobe and the posterior lobe, leaving the other lateral lobe for a further resection at a later date. It is surprising on these occasions that the patient may succeed in passing urine even before the other lobe is resected.

Assuming no obesity and a healthy cardio-respiratory system, the guiding factor is a prostate somewhere around 25 g.

In other words, a prostate over 30 g would normally be removed by retropubic prostatectomy, while an adenoma of less than 20 g would always be resected. In the training of a urologist, it is important to ensure that he is equally capable of carrying out a retropubic prostatectomy as well as a transurethral resection and under no circumstances should his choice of operation be guided by any limitation of his surgical skill at either of these operations. This leaves the 20–30 g adenoma which represents the overlap between open surgery and transurethral resection, where both methods are possible and reasonable (Mitchell[30]).

Nothing is achieved to the advantage of the patient in attempting to remove adenomata of more than 30 g by the transurethral route.

CONTRA-INDICATIONS

Various factors may make transurethral resection either difficult or dangerous. For example, a urethral stricture would be aggravated by the presence of a resectoscope in the urethra for a period of approximately one hour, while evidence of urethritis would present an increased risk of bacteremia or even septicemia from the constant irritation of the urethra by the resectoscope sheath.

Occasionally, an attempt at transurethral resection has to be abandoned because of the development of priapism. This not only makes the manipulation of the instrument difficult and increases the risk of stricture formation, but also the associated hyperemia of the bladder neck during the episode of priapism will result in excessive bleeding. In a fully developed priapism, a resectoscope of normal length will not even reach the prostate and bladder neck, so that resection is impossible.

As with urethritis, an acute cystitis is a contra-indication to immediate transurethral resection, and a period of bladder drainage, treatment with antibiotics and perhaps instillation of an antiseptic solution, will prepare the patient for transurethral surgery at a later date.

The size of the bladder can occasionally influence one's decision regarding the mode of approach. A bladder of small capacity will not allow sufficient irrigating fluid to enter the bladder, and the surgeon will find that he spends far too much time emptying the bladder and reorientating himself to make transurethral resection a practical proposition. However, as we know, a bladder of small capacity can be an extreme embarrassment even at open surgery and the patient will have post-operative problems of bladder spasm, contracting down onto the balloon of the catheter. A bladder of a capacity of less than 250 ml can be an embarrassment for transurethral resection, though the operation may still be possible. When the capacity is reduced to 100 ml or less, then transurethral resection is virtually impossible, as the time of orientation before any operative procedure will consume most of the flow of the irrigating fluid allowed by such a limited volume.

Physical deformities of the hip joints and lower limbs can create a problem at transurethral resection. The patient with a slightly flexed adducted thigh will make access to the lobe of the prostate on the contra-lateral side very difficult, if not impossible. However, provided that there is some degree of flexion of the hip joint, with a corresponding lordosis of the lumbar spine, it may be possible for the surgeon to work below

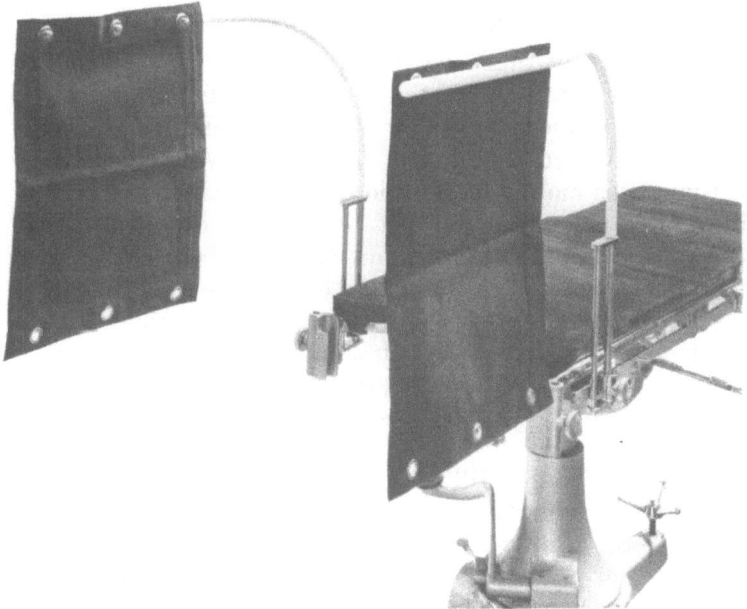

Figure 3.2   Leg Stirrups (By courtesy of Thackrays, Leeds, England)

the legs, even in those patients who have a bilateral fixed hip. Careful positioning of the patient in suitable leg stirrups can[31] improve what would otherwise be an impossible situation (Figure 3.2).

Associated pathology in the bladder can modify the timing of a transurethral resection. It has been found (Miller, Mitchell and Brown[32]) that resection of the bladder tumor and the bladder neck and prostate at the same operation does not appear to increase the risk of implantation of seedlings from the tumor onto the bare area of the prostatic bed. On the other hand, the association of calculi and a diverticulum usually demands a two-stage operation, particularly in the presence of infection. It is my experience that litholapaxy, when followed by transurethral resection, is more often associated with post-operative complications of infection, hemorrhage and slow convalescence, than when the two procedures are carried out at an interval of at least a week. The diverticulum can be removed by open surgery two weeks after the transurethral resection.

HYPOTENSIVE ANESTHESIA

Hypotensive anesthesia has given dramatic improvement in the management of the benign adenoma of the prostate by transurethral resection, as well as by retropubic prostatectomy. A well balanced anesthetic with a steady hypotension is perhaps even more important in transurethral surgery than in retropubic prostatectomy. The blood pressure that oscillates can cause alarming bleeding one minute and the next minute there is insufficient evidence of bleeding points to be able to be satisfied that the area has been adequately controlled. If the surgeon is uncertain of his anesthetist colleague's ability to maintain a steady hypotension, then he is well advised to adopt a safer procedure of normotensive anesthesia.

THE RESECTOSCOPE

Numerous modifications have been made on the original design by Stern and McCarthy[27,28], though little change in the angle of view of the telescope has been made, with the exception of a few instruments constructed around the direct vision telescope (Mitchell[26]). Various designs are on the market,

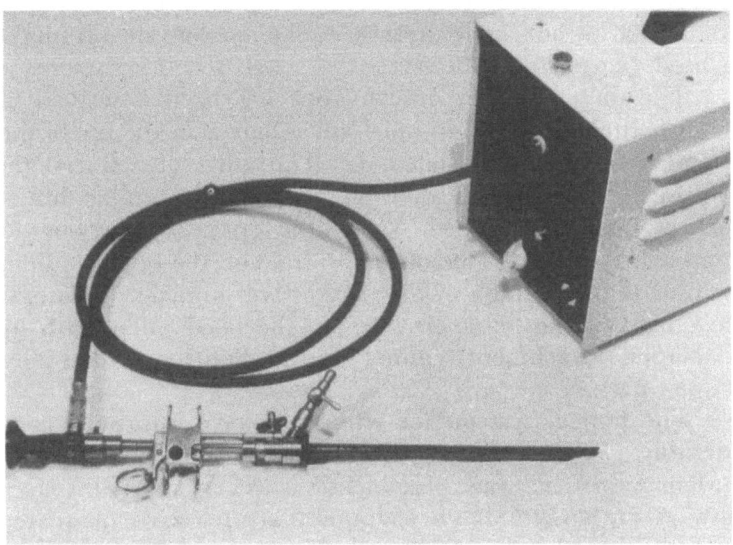

Figure 3.3 The author's resectoscope. From *The Principles of Transurethral Resection and Haemostatis*. (By courtesy of John Wright, Bristol, England)

most of which work on the principle of a recoil spring, the resting position of which may, in some designs, hold the loop protected in the sheath, but in other designs, the rest position may leave the loop dangerously situated beyond the sheath itself, where accidental activation of the diathermy could result in a perforation. Some designs rely on the movement of the thumb, others use a movable carriage, operated by the fore-finger and middle finger. Yet other designs have a scissor-grip action or pistol grip. The resectoscope illustrated (Figure 3.3) (Mitchell[33,34]) here has no spring and the carriage runs on nylon roller bearings. The object of this modification is to give better tactile sensibility of the movement of the loop and its contact with the tissues. The exact amount of pressure being exerted between the loop and the tissues to be cut is not masked by the presence of a recoil spring.

The water inlet is angled away from the operator and is on a rotatable collar.

The diathermy socket on the carriage can be changed from side to side as the instrument is rotated. The size of the sheath varies from 24 to 26. Just occasionally, in a capacious urethra, or in the female urethra, a 28 Charrière sheath might be used, but this must be rare.

The direct viewing resectoscope has been described in detail (Mitchell[26]) and its chief advantage is in the use of the direct vision fiber-light telescope. The pillar of a fiber-light telescope is at present fixed, as no satisfactory rotatable design has yet been constructed. When the operator is trying to approach the lateral lobe of the prostate on the opposite side, he finds that the thigh of the patient will impede the lateral movement of the telescope because the fixed pillar with its fiber-light attachment cannot move sufficiently laterally (Figure 3.4).

The optical systems for telescopes have improved considerably over the last five years (Hopkins[35]). By constructing the lens system in a series of rod lenses with very short air spaces between the lenses, it has been found that a telescope of greater resolution and increased light transmission can be produced. This solid rod lens system, associated with the development of fibre illumination has vastly improved the quality of transurethral techniques. Unfortunately, at present there has been little success in attempts to standardize the fiber-light cables and the fittings of the pillar to which they are attached.

Sterilization of these instruments can be carried out by immersion in a sterilizing fluid, enclosure in a disinfecting vapor, or by low pressure steam with or without formaldehyde. Of these methods hibitane 0.5% in 70% spirit is the quickest and most effective sterilizing fluid, but care must be taken to ensure that the instrument is never left in this fluid for more than the required time of two minutes, otherwise serious damage will occur to the cement of the lens mounting. Gluteraldehyde (Cidex) is also an effective method of cold sterilization but, unfortunately, the solution gives off a pungent smell, very much akin to formalin. In Bristol low pressure steam has now been used for over ten years. This has to be carefully controlled to ensure that the temperature does not rise above 80 °C and the manufacturers must be warned that although at 80 °C steam only requires half an atmosphere of decompression, nevertheless the instrument should be capable of withstanding pressures down to an eighth or a tenth of an atmosphere during

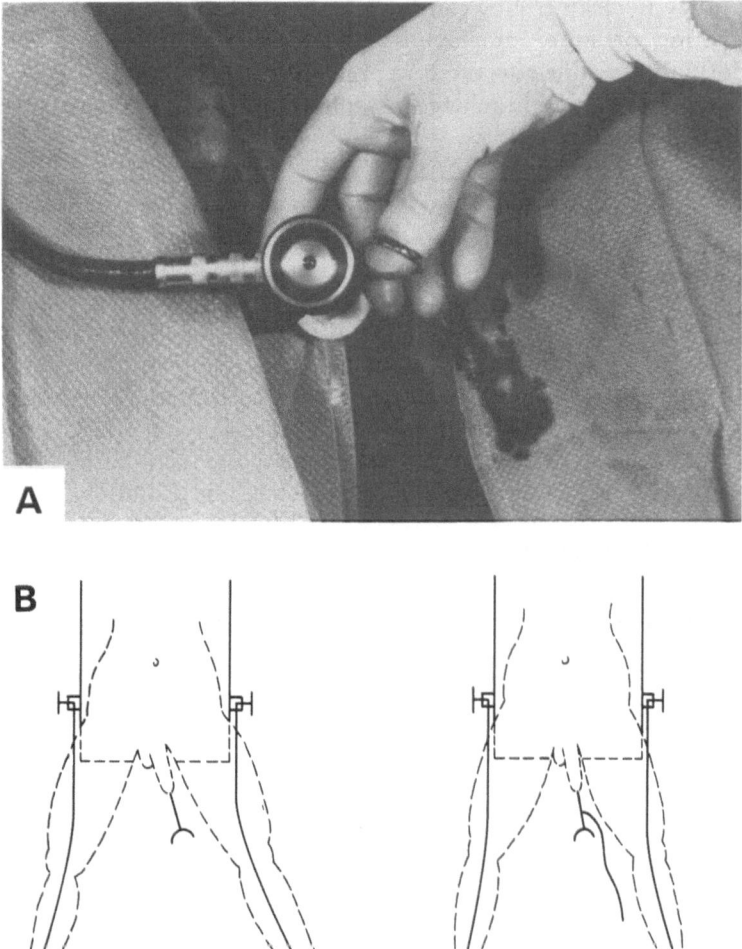

Figure 3.4   The limitation of lateral movement as a result of the fixed fiber-light pillar. (A) View from above; (B) Diagramatic view. From *The Principles of Transurethral Resection and Haemostasis*. (By courtesy of John Wright, Bristol, England)

the evacuation stage of the cycle. Careful monitoring must ensure that in no circumstances, does the cycle take the temperature above 80 °C. This process using low pressure steam provides a disinfected instrument, ready for use, in a sterile box and therefore fits admirably with the organization of a theatre sterile supply unit. The turn round time from dirty trolley to clean trolley can be as little as 18 minutes, provided the low pressure autoclave is not too far from the theater. If formalin is added to the low pressure steam cycle then complete sterilization is achieved (Alder, Gingell and Mitchell[36]).

THE DIATHERMY MACHINE

A diathermy providing two circuits, namely a valve circuit and a spark gap or spark gap-simulated circuit, is essential for transurethral resection. Electrosection is slow, of poor quality, and the cut tissue sticks to the electrode if the spark gap is used for cutting. The higher frequency provided by a valve machine will give sharp dissection, relatively little reaction in the tissues around and no adherence of the necrotic tissue to the electrode. Conversely, coagulation is best achieved by a spark gap diathermy. Hence the need to have a machine with both valve and spark gap circuits available (Mitchell and Lumb[37]).

THE TECHNIQUE

The first and most essential features in the technique of transurethral resection are, first to achieve good hemostasis and,

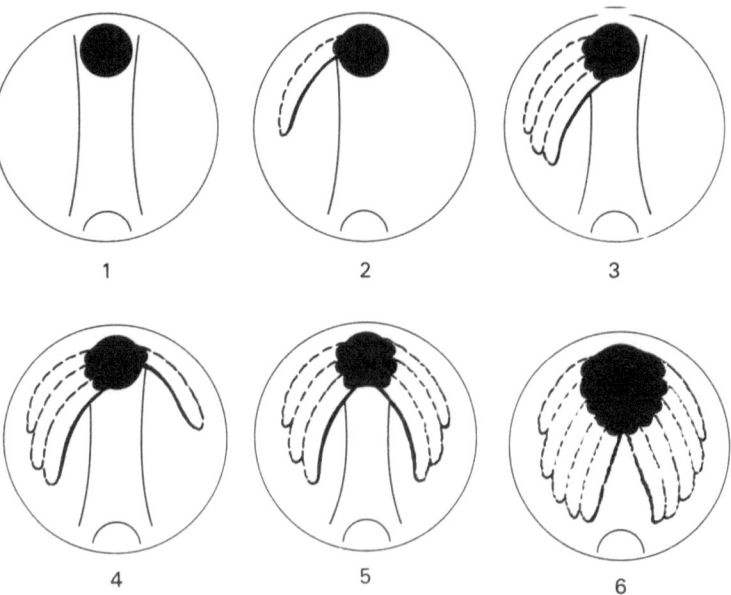

Figure 3.5   The stages of transurethral resection of prostate and bladder neck

secondly, quick orientation. Once these two skills have been acquired, the process of resection becomes less hazardous and less alarming for the surgeon.

Most resectionists begin either at the 11 o'clock or 1 o'clock position. The object of the resection should be to cut a channel between the adenoma and the capsule (Figure 3.5). The capsule can be recognized by ring-like muscle fibers at the bladder neck. Lower down the prostatic urethra these muscle fibers appear to criss-cross, again giving a characteristic appearance. As the dissection by the loop electrode proceeds the lateral lobe falls downwards and medially. When the resection reaches 8 o'clock or 4 o'clock large vessels are usually encountered and these should be controlled by coagulation immediately. The opposite lobe is then treated in a similar manner and, finally, the middle lobe is resected down to the bladder neck. Having completed these stages the apex of each lobe is resected down to, or adjacent to the verumontanum. The apical lobes must be resected *in toto*, as otherwise they are liable to cause obstruction by a ball valve action into the area of the external sphincter. Needless to say, the surgeon must take extreme care to ensure that he does not encroach on the area of the external sphincter as the slightest damage in this area with a resectoscope will result in total, permanent incontinence post-operatively.

Immediate complications of transurethral resection
Perforation is the immediate complication which seems to create the most anxiety, but it can be recognized without delay, from the deterioration in the patient's general condition or abdominal tenderness as he comes round from the anesthetic. Preferably it should be spotted, at the time the perforation occurs, by the 'cobwebby' appearance between the muscle fibres which have been perforated. A perforation which has caused sufficient extravasation to present with abdominal pain post-operatively should be drained with a suprapubic drain passed into the extra-vesical area. On the other hand, a minute perforation, if spotted immediately, may be treated by simple catheter drainage, having discontinued the resection from the time the perforation occurs.

One of the commonest causes of perforation in the area of

11 o'clock or 1 o'clock is damage to the midline where there is little prostatic tissue as a result of deflection of the midline at the time the first lobe is resected (Mitchell[30]).

Hemorrhage at the time of operation can be a tiresome and tedious problem. The resectionist is well advised to ensure that he coagulates every major bleeding vessel as soon as it is encountered. It can be very tempting to leave a bleeding vessel on the assumption that it will easily be controlled later. However, much valuable time can be lost in trying to orientate when a second vessel has been cut and bleeding is occurring into the face of the lens from two different directions.

Cutting the trigone
It is very easy to make the mistake of resecting down the trigone, which is a highly vascular area. This mistake is usually made due to the instrument being held too near to the neck of the bladder (Figure 3.6). If the sheath is retracted down the urethra so that the extended loop just reaches the bladder neck, then there is little risk of creeping down the trigone and causing embarrassing hemorrhage.

Finally, the chippings are evacuated from the bladder by means of a glass bulb evacuator.

The irrigating fluid should be delivered at no more than 60 cm of water pressure and near isotonic solutions of either sugar or glycine should be available during the resection before the loop is approaching the capsular vessels. The reason for these two precautions is to ensure a minimum amount of irrigating fluid being absorbed into the exposed prostatic venous sinuses. With the patient in the lithotomy position it is possible that many of these venous sinuses are at a very low positive pressure and if the patient is tilted head down, it is quite probable that these vessels will, in fact, be at a negative pressure. Consequently if fluid is delivered at a high pressure and is not isotonic, then there is a serious risk of hemolysis occurring with possible renal failure. In addition to delivering at a maximum pressure of 60 cm H_2O, and in isotonic solution, a non-return valve must be inserted in the circuit so that if the patient does contract his abdominal muscles during the operation, then fluid from the patient's bladder will not pass retrogradely up the irrigating tube into the reservoir, thus contaminating the reservoir jar.

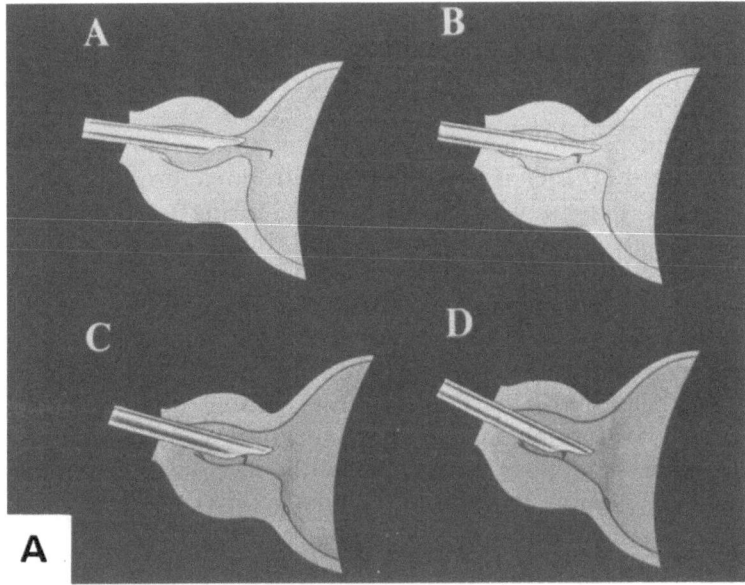

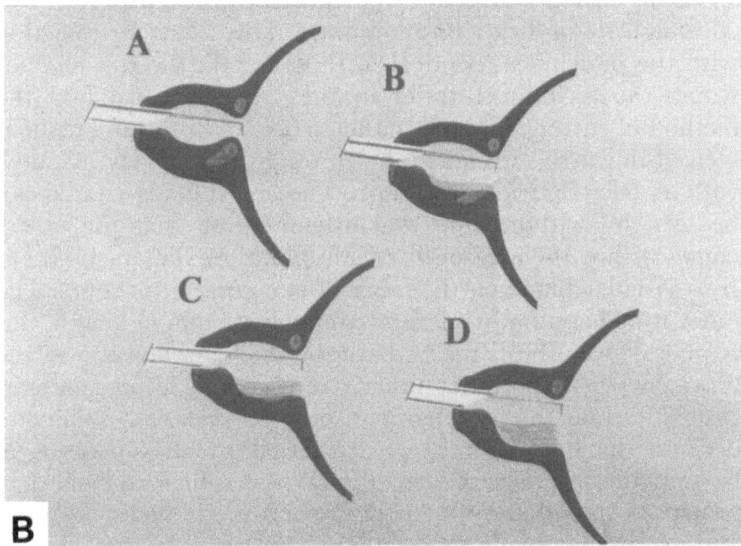

Figure 3.6 (A) Ineffective resection of the bladder neck posteriorly by 'creeping' down the trigone; (B) Correcting the line of cut by withdrawing the resectoscope down the urethra, to avoid 'creeping' down the trigone. From *The Principles of Transurethral Resection and Haemostasis*. (By courtesy of John Wright, Bristol, England)

If the urethra is narrow, there should be no hesitation in performing either an internal urethrotomy or a perineal urethrotomy in order to introduce the instrument (see page 79 of this text).

The patient should then be put onto a closed circuit catheter drainage, as described for retropubic prostatectomy.

The patient who bleeds heavily during operation will usually give trouble with clots and bleeding in the post-operative stage. It is, therefore, wise to take the precaution of having blood available if blood has been needed during operation.

Post-operative complications of transurethral resection are either from hemorrhage or from cutting when not satis-factorily orientated. Damage to the prostatic capsule can result in perforation, while cutting below the level of the verumon-tanum can injure the external sphincter with consequent post-operative incontinence.

Transurethral resection by the Thompson punch

Although the indications and contra-indications for resection with the punch are identical to those for the electric resecto-scope, the techniques differ in the view obtained and the method of cutting. There is no telescope and prostatic tissue is viewed down the straight tube through a clear glass window with no telescopic magnification. The object being viewed can be seen by withdrawing the instrument so that the object comes within the area of distal illumination. The tissue is cut by a circular blade on the inner of two concentric tubes. The outer tube has a foramen approximately 15 mm in length, this is placed over the tissue to be cut, which prolapses into the foramen when the inner tube is retracted. This tissue, as it protrudes into the foramen, can only be seen as a silhouette because the light source, when viewed by the operator, is beyond the foramen of the tube. When sufficient tissue has prolapsed into the foramen the inner tube is thrust forward and its circular blade slices off the prolapsing tissue. After a few cuts the area is again viewed by withdrawing the instru-ment so that the cut area is illuminated by the distal light and can be seen through the distal end of the instrument. Bleeding points can then be coagulated by a button electrode which is passed down the electrode channel.

The principle of the procedure is very similar to that used with the electric resectoscope in that the operator starts at either 11 o'clock or 1 o'clock, cuts in depth will then expose the circular fibers of the bladder neck and the criss-cross fibers of the prostatic capsule; from then on the operator cuts between capsule and adenoma, so that the adenoma falls medially. At about 4 o'clock or 8 o'clock, depending on which side is being cut, the major vessels passing through at the level of the bladder neck will be exposed, and these can be controlled by coagulation. After these vessels have been controlled, resection of the two lateral lobes and middle lobe is relatively avascular. Finally, the apical lobe on each side is resected.

Although it is an advantage for surgeons to be trained in the use of both the electric resectoscope and the punch, this is today perhaps an ideal which is too time consuming for the limited experience that a trainee can cover in the time permitted. So much training is necessary in other aspects of urology, that it is generally accepted today that trainees will learn one or other procedure. 80–90% of urological clinics now use the electric resectoscope and less than 20% still use the punch.

The only modifications that have occurred on the punch in recent years have been attempts to construct a single-handed rotatable instrument[38]. The punch is still approximately 27 Charrière, as compared with 26 or even 24 Charrière for the electric resectoscope, consequently there is an increased risk of stricture formation post-operatively, simply from the larger calibre of the instrument itself.

Urethrotomy and meatotomy

Occasionally the urethra is found to be tight to the instrument. The tightness may be localized to the external meatus, or the base of the navicular fossa, in which case a meatotomy is required. This should be a generous cut to a distance of 1 cm proximal to the base of the navicular fossa. The orifice will close down to some extent, but the patient must be warned that his stream is liable to spray and he will have to learn the technique for holding the penis in order to avoid the embarrassment of spraying urine down his trouser front.

If the tightness of the urethra seems to be through the entire length, then the operator has a choice of either a urethrotomy, using an Otis urethrotome, or a perineal urethrotomy. It is very rare that any tightness is encountered from the region of the bulb proximally and by opening the bulbous urethra the 26 or 27 Charrière instrument can be passed relatively easily. Closure of the perineal urethrotomy usually occurs without any problem, though the patient may have a little more pain passing water when the catheter is removed in the early stages. Although internal urethrotomy is a simple procedure, it does carry certain risks of heavy bleeding, subsequent stricture formation and even occasionally a postoperative chordee. For these reasons I prefer a perineal urethrotomy, which is a simple procedure and takes little longer than an internal urethrotomy.

Retropubic prostatectomy
As already described (see page 68 of this book) the indications for retropubic prostatectomy as opposed to transurethral resection are purely a matter of size of the adenoma. An adenoma of 30 g or more will enucleate readily, provided there is no neoplastic change. The size of 30 g is a very arbitrary figure in that the surgeon should take into account certain other factors, such as the size of the patient, his cardio-respiratory condition and any other clinical complicating factors. In an obese patient a gland estimated to be a little more than 30 g would still be attempted by transurethral resection. Similarly, a patient with cardio-respiratory limitation who has an adenomatous gland of 40–50 g in size could have a lower operative risk by transurethral resection than by open prostatectomy.

All patients will have a routine midstream specimen of urine sent for deposit and culture. An intravenous pyelogram is a routine investigation for all candidates for prostatectomy under the age of 75. Over the age of 75 it is considered that the incidental finding of any renal pathology, which in itself had produced no symptoms, would probably not be followed up surgically and, therefore, the radiological investigation in these patients is limited to a straight x-ray of abdomen and pelvis. In order to assess renal function, however, it is advisable that a blood urea estimation should be made.

A preliminary cystoscopy should be performed in all patients only as a pre-operative investigation at the time of prostatectomy, in order to exclude any intra-vesical pathology and to confirm the route of approach (i.e. transurethral resection or retropubic). To carry out a cystoscopy several days beforehand cannot be justified today, as this does not help in deciding whether or not to operate and increases the risk of pre-operative infection. The decision to proceed with prostatectomy will already have been made on the patient's symptoms and signs and the result of his intravenous pyelogram.

The patient is laid on the table in the supine position with approximately 20–25° of Trendelenburg tilt. The towels are draped so that there can be access to the external genitalia for instrumentation of the urethra and in order to perform transscrotal vasotomy if this is considered necessary at the end of the operation. The draping drill recommended is to leave the genitalia and lower abdomen exposed, clipping a small extra towel across the lower part of the operative area, so that this can be folded downward over the genitalia. This flap can then be raised when access to the external meatus is necessary for the passage of a catheter (see Figure 3.7).

The prostate can be approached either via a vertical midline suprapubic incision or via a transverse incision one inch above the symphysis pubis in the line of the skin creases. In the latter case the aponeurosis is also divided transversely and the recti are then exposed and retracted, the aponeurosis having been dissected upwards and downwards from the surface of the recti muscles. There has been much discussion regarding the pros and cons of these two incisions. It is thought that the vertical incision is more likely to result in a ventral hernia, but this can usually be traced to one of two causes: either inadequate suturing of the wound or, more likely, infection. On the other hand, the transverse incision lies in the natural fold of the abdominal wall when the patient is in the sitting position, and if there is any obesity the transverse incision will be buried in the skin fold and, consequently, is very liable to become

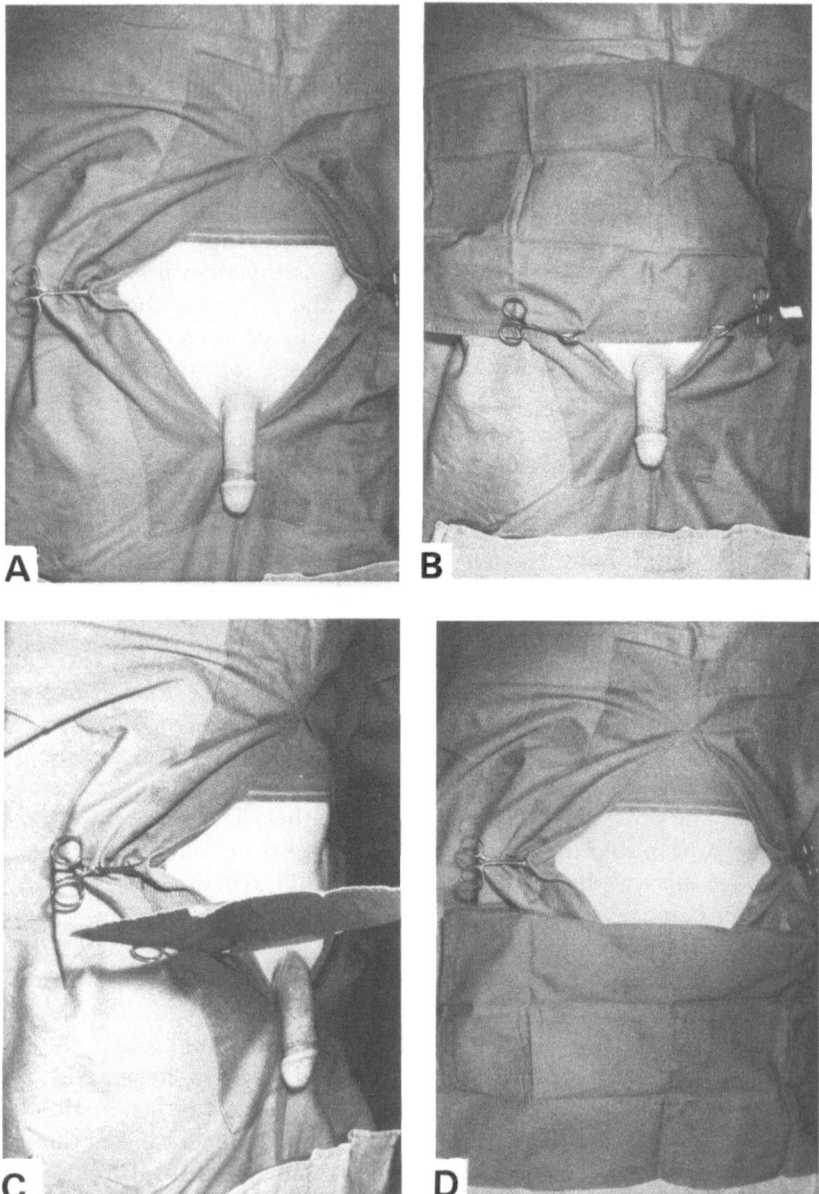

Figure 3.7 (A), (B), (C), (D)   Stages in draping the patient preparatory to retropubic prostatectomy

macerated, hence aggravating the risk of infection of the wound. I have seen a ventral hernia following a transverse as well as a vertical incision. Finally, the vertical incision does give a little better exposure.

The Millin's retractors with two different lengths of blade for patients of variable obesity is inserted after separating the tissues digitally. This digital dissection should extend laterally on either side of the bladder so as to give a good exposure of the whole of the anterior surface of the bladder, and the fingers should then be passed downwards behind the symphysis pubis so as to separate all the areolar tissue in front and on either side of the prostate and bladder neck. This separation should be performed as gently as possible to avoid tearing any veins of the pre-prostatic plexus, and it should extend downwards as far as the anterior prostatic ligaments which run from the lower border of the prostate to the lower part of the posterior aspect of the symphysis pubis just above the medial fibres of the levator ani. This separation of the tissues anterior to the prostate and behind the symphysis pubis is an essential part of retropubic prostatectomy, because only after separation of these tissues can the prostate be hinged backwards on its apex so as to give an adequate exposure of its anterior surface. In the majority of occasions when the statement has been made that 'a retropubic prostatectomy is an awkward operation' the reason is usually failure to mobilize and hinge the prostate backwards (see Figure 3.8). Occasionally fibrosis in this area from any previous operative intervention may be so dense as to make digital separation impossible and knife dissection is the only practical approach.

If, at this stage, it is found that the bladder has still retained some fluid, even though a preliminary endoscopy was carried out, then the bladder must be emptied. Again, the prostate will not hinge back into the pelvis satisfactorily if the bladder still contains a certain amount of fluid. To remove this fluid a wide bore needle on the end of the sucker can be passed through the anterior wall of the bladder.

The collapsed bladder is held backwards by the centre blade of Millin's retractor and the bladder neck area is pushed backwards by means of two sponge-holding forceps loaded

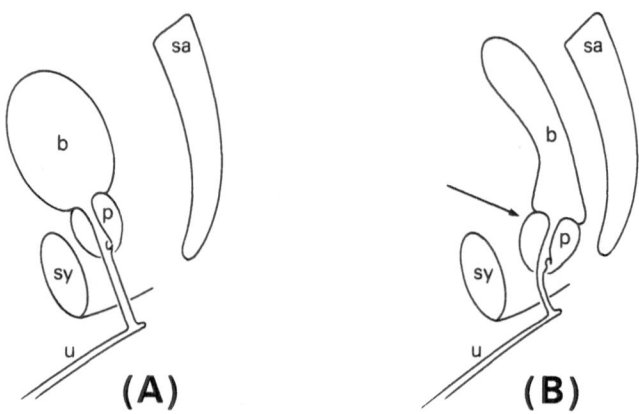

Figure 3.8   Hingeing the prostate backwards. (A) shows the bladder full; (B) shows the bladder empty, the prostate hinged backwards and the approach in the line of the arrow.   u = anterior   urethra,   sy = symphysis   pubis,   p = prostate,   b = bladder, sa = sacrum

with swabs, which press downwards and backwards on either side of the bladder neck.

The anterior surface of the prostate must now be cleared, carefully avoiding puncturing or tearing the veins which course across in the preprostatic plexus. These veins can be large and, if torn, may cause troublesome bleeding. The commonest distribution is two main veins which run up from the lower part of the pre-prostatic plexus upwards and outwards on the anterior surface of the prostate. These can be picked up with forceps and ligated. Usually these veins are too large and surrounded by too much fat to coagulate with diathermy.

Having exposed the anterior surface of the prostate two stay sutures are inserted and tied. A transverse incision is then made at the junction of the lower two-thirds and upper third — in other words usually at the level about 1–2 cm below the neck of the bladder and between the two stay sutures. This transverse incision should be a generous incision extending to nearly half the circumference of the prostate. Fairly heavy bleeding will be encountered from the vessels lying in the layers of the capsule of the prostate. These, however, can be readily diathermized; the largest ones will be found in the midline anteriorly and will probably have already been occluded by the two stay sutures. A further large vessel will be found about 1 cm on either side of the midline, and often another large vessel will be cut at the lateral limits of the incision in the capsule. Again, these will all usually be controlled readily with diathermy coagulation. The incision is carried deep enough to expose the full width of the adenoma, which appears as a distinctly different amorphous tissue as compared to the fibromuscular layers of the capsule.

Enucleation of the adenoma should not start until all vessels in the capsular incision and all pre-prostatic veins have been satisfactorily ligated or coagulated. By this stage a bloodless field should have been achieved, with the additional help of the hypotensive anesthesia. Enucleation is then started by blunt dissection with the blades of the long curved scissors (Nelson Roberts). These are passed down between the capsule and adenoma at the lateral limits of the capsular incision on either side, and the blades are then separated. Similarly, the enucleation is continued with the scissors upwards between the adenoma and the neck of the bladder on either side of the midline, and downwards toward the apex of the prostate between the adenoma and the capsule on either side of the midline. When this separation has been carried out with the scissors, as much as two-thirds of the enucleation will have been performed. The remaining part of the enucleation is completed with the tip of the finger of the right hand. Great care must be taken (1) not to drag up the mucosa from the membranous urethra and (2) to keep well toward the adenoma in the layer between the adenoma and capsule, even at the expense, perhaps, of erring on the side of removing too little rather than too much. It is within this posterior part of the capsule that the venous plexus of Santorini lies, and it is liable to be damaged by the enucleating finger tip if this is allowed to dig too deeply into the lower posterior part of the capsule of the gland. Profuse and uncontrollable bleeding from the posterior part of the apex of the prostatic cavity is the price of such rough enucleation. The enucleating finger must work gently and must feel accurately the plane of cleavage around the adenoma.

Care with enucleation in this area can considerably reduce the amount of bleeding after enucleation. If any difficulty is encountered breaking through the urethral mucosa at the apex of the prostate, then this should be divided by scissor dissection. If too much adenomatous tissue has been left in the region of the apex of the prostatic cavity in an effort to avoid damage to the capsule and bleeding from the plexus of Santorini, then this can easily be dissected later in the operation. The adenoma of prostate is then delivered through the incision in the anterior part of the capsule, though it is still attached in the region of the neck of the bladder.

With volsellum forceps the adenoma is then lifted into the wound, drawing up the neck of the bladder, which can easily be seen for scissor dissection. It is at this stage that a bladder neck spreader is invaluable[39] (see Figure 3.9). The blades of the spreader are inserted into the neck of the bladder and these can be opened or relaxed as seems most convenient at the various stages of dissection of the bladder neck. At 4 o'clock

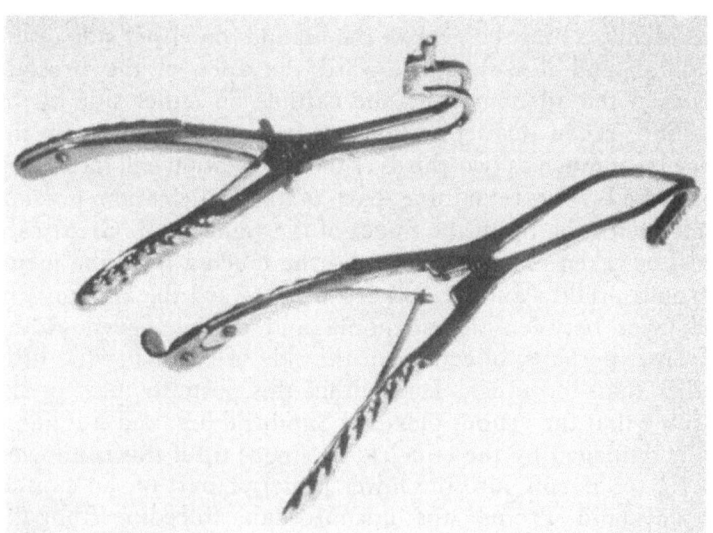

Figure 3.9 Bladder neck spreader. (From Mitchell, 1952, by courtesy of *Lancet*, *1*, 193)

and 8 o'clock large vessels will be encountered as the bladder neck is dissected, and these can be caught in the tip of the Nelson Roberts forceps and diathermized directly.

A word of warning is appropriate at this stage not to pick up too large a bite of tissue in the Nelson Roberts forceps. If only the vessel itself is caught in the forceps then adequate coagulation can be obtained by white fulguration. There is no need to use the diathermy excessively to the extent of black coagulation[37] which inevitably leaves a much larger area of necrotic tissue and consequently an increased risk of infection and secondary hemorrhage.

Despite careful diathermy coagulation of bleeding vessels at the neck of the bladder, a considerable amount of bleeding may still occur either from part of the prostatic capsule or at the neck of the bladder.

At the same time as dissecting the adenoma from the neck of the bladder, a good crescent of tissue from the neck itself should be dissected, taking almost the entire posterior half of the internal sphincter, having previously identified both ureteric orifices. At the end of this resection it should be possible to introduce two fingers comfortably into the bladder neck beyond their proximal interphalangeal joints. At the same time the cavity of the bladder is palpated to ensure that no loose fragment of adenoma has been dislocated upwards, possibly hanging by a strand of urethra, or even lying free within the bladder.

Finally, the cavity of the prostate is examined by palpation with the finger and by direct inspection, to ensure that no isolated adenoma has been left adhering to the capsule. The next stage is a figure-of-eight ligation at 8 o'clock and 4 o'clock. This is easy to insert with the boomerang needle and is illustrated in Figure 3.10. The lower stitch takes in the capsule of the prostate, the posterior part of the neck of the bladder and the proximal part of the bladder wall. The second part of the stitch merely passes through the prostatic capsule and the neck of the bladder. After tying this stitch on each side there is a dramatic reduction in the amount of oozing. When this stage has been completed, the field should be virtually bloodless, unless damage has occurred to the capsule and plexus of Santorini in the posterior part of the apex of the prostate. This

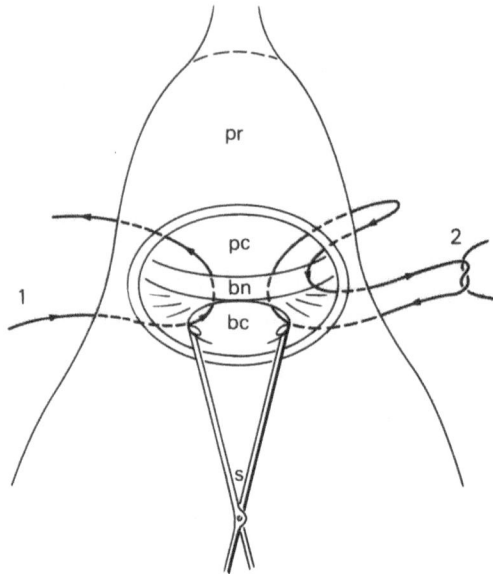

Figure 3.10 Suture inserted at 4 o'clock and 8 o'clock at the bladder neck to give partial obliteration of the prostatic cavity and hemostasis of the major arterial supply in this area. The suture should be of absorbable material. (1) shows the first part of the figure-of-eight suture and (2) shows the ligation complete and ready to be tied. pr, prostatic capsule; pc, prostatic cavity; bn, bladder neck; bc, bladder cavity; s, bladder neck spreader

stitch also obliterates part of the prostatic cavity, because the laterally inserted part of each of these stitches passes through the prostatic capsule well down toward the apex. Hence, when the stitch is tied, part of the prostatic capsule is collapsed and the effect is comparable to Harris's original suture, which has subsequently been referred to as the 're-trigonizing stitch', but could more appropriately be called the 'hemostatic and cavity obliterating stitch'.

An 18 or 20 Charrière balloon catheter (Foley type) is passed *per urethram* after instillation of 5 ml of 0·5% Chlorhexidine (hibitane) in glycerine to avoid carrying any organisms from the distal urethra into the prostatic cavity. The incision in the prostatic capsule is closed by suturing with the boomerang needle and a retropubic drain is placed between the symphysis pubis and the anterior surface of the prostate.

Transvesical prostatectomy

Occasionally pathology within the bladder, which the surgeon may wish to remove at the same time as the operation of prostatectomy, will demand a transvesical approach. For example, a diverticulum, a small neoplasm of bladder, or a large calculus could influence the surgeon into making this alternative approach. Otherwise transvesical prostatectomy is rarely performed today in urological clinics. Hemostasis is less reliable because all parts of the prostatic cavity are less clearly exposed, and consequently the post-operative catheter has to remain *in situ* for a longer period, usually around 5 days, as opposed to 2 days with retropubic prostatectomy.

For these reasons the operation of transvesical prostatectomy will only be described in brief. If a stone is too large to remove through the neck of the bladder at the time of retropubic prostatectomy, then the bladder neck can always be divided for a short distance anteriorly to extract the stone. Diverticulae are much more common in association with the small fibrous prostate and bladder neck obstruction than with the large adenomatous prostate. In these cases it is preferable to remove the diverticulum and the prostate at two separate operations, the prostate being resected by the transurethral route. Only when a large diverticulum or a moderate-sized bladder tumor, treatable by open resection and diathermy is associated with adenomatous enlargement of the prostate would I use a transvesical approach.

The bladder is opened by a vertical incision, which is extended upward rather than toward the neck of the bladder. This will necessitate separation of the peritoneum from the vault and part of the posterior wall of the bladder, where in fact it is most adherent due to the fibrous remnant of the urachus. If the opening of the bladder is not extended upward, then the viscus cannot be retracted into a spherical shape and the posterior wall of the bladder beyond the trigone forms a large lax fold, which can be inconvenient and obstruct part of the field during the operation. If the bladder wall is opened upward, then the Morson bladder retractor, when inserted into the cavity, will open the bladder into a completely spherical shape, obliterating this transverse posterior fold in the bladder base.

The mucosa over the posterior part of the middle lobe and both lateral lobes is divided by a diathermy cutting needle in a crescentic incision, extending from one lateral lobe, across the middle lobe to the opposite lateral lobe taking a crescent of internal sphincter until the adenomatous tissue is exposed. Enucleation is carried out by a finger passed down between the adenomatous tissue and the capsule, breaking through the urethra cleanly at the apex of the prostate and ensuring that no urethral mucosa is drawn up from the membranous urethra. If any doubt exists regarding the completeness of the break through in the urethral mucosa at the apex, this should be divided with scissors. Unfortunately, it is almost impossible to do this under direct vision in the depths of the prostatic cavity, and the tips of the scissor blades have to be guided accurately in the line of the enucleating finger.

Every effort at hemostasis must be made at this stage. Similar sutures at 4 o'clock and 8 o'clock to those already described under retropubic prostatectomy should be inserted to control the major vessels of the bladder neck. A large hemostatic suture in the anterior wall of the prostatic capsule can help to control the major vessels passing in this area. An indwelling catheter of size 20 or 22 Charrière (a little larger than that used for retropubic prostatectomy) will be necessary to drain the bladder. After closure of the bladder a retropubic drain is left *in situ*.

Catheter management after prostatectomy

It has been shown that the management of the post-operative catheter can reduce considerably the incidence of infection following prostatectomy[40,41,42]. A closed system of drainage is set up in the operating theater, with or without irrigation. The catheter must be introduced in the theater and checked before the drainage system is connected to ensure that there is a free flow and no residual clot remaining in the bladder to obstruct the eye of the catheter. From then on the drainage system should not be disconnected for any purpose except a major clot retention. Disconnection of the closed drainage system will almost inevitably result in contamination and infection of the urine and subsequently the prostatic bed.

The catheter must be anchored so that there is no drag

whatever on the urethra. Tapes around the catheter are pinned to a piece of Elastoplast on the thigh (Figure 3.11). This detachable anchorage allows freedom for nursing care but, at the same time, it ensures a firm anchorage of the drainage tube.

The external meatus will be found to accumulate a certain amount of discharge around the catheter. This is a foreign body reaction and will be proportionate to the size of the catheter. The discharge should be cleansed with a detergent solution such as Cetavlon or Cetrimide, the catheter should be exposed for a distance of 1 centimeter by retracting the penis, and the area of catheter around the meatus then smeared with a small quantity of chlorhexidine cream. The penis is then allowed to slide down the catheter once again, over the cream. This toilet to the external meatus should be carried out every 12 hours, so long as the catheter is indwelling[43].

The irrigation system (Figure 3.12) shows the use of a Higginson's bulb in the outflow of the drainage, which allows some aspiration of the catheter by suction. The scheme of drainage is well described elsewhere[26]. It is important to ensure that the nurse understands the irrigation system, otherwise there is a serious risk that she may, in her efforts to clear the catheter, distend the bladder with air, causing considerable distress to the patient and the possible risk of air embolus. It is essential that the nurse is certain she has filled the Higginson's bulb with irrigating fluid before compression, otherwise she can aspirate air from the drainage bag or bottle.

Any distension of the bladder will stretch the prostatic cavity and, in turn, open up vessels which have been sealed

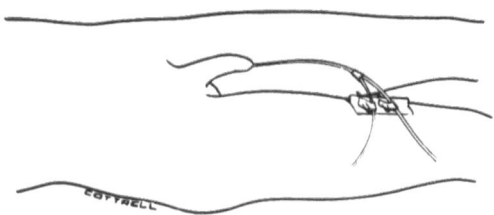

Figure 3.11 Anchoring an indwelling catheter by means of Elastoplast and safety pins. From *The Principles of Transurethral Resection and Haemostasis*. (By courtesy of John Wright, Bristol, England)

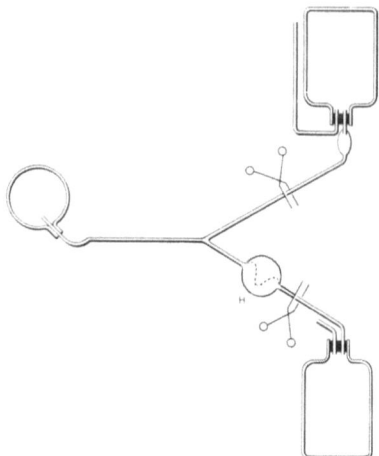

Figure 3.12   Closed drainage system with irrigation. H = Higginson syringe balloon.
From 'Urology for Nurses'. (By courtesy of John Wright, Bristol, England)

with blood clots and coagulated with diathermy. If the bladder
is allowed to distend through inadequate observation in the
immediate post-operative stage, this will certainly aggravate
further bleeding. Careful observation of the catheter in the
early post-operative stage is such a vital factor in the management of prostatectomy that it is advisable for the surgeon to
ensure that all the nursing staff on the route from theater to
ward are well trained in this discipline. If the patient is being
returned via the recovery ward, it is possible that the nursing
staff in that department may not have had a full urological
training and may be uncertain of the management of catheter
drainage. Once the patient returns to the urological ward, he
will be under the care of fully trained urological staff, and the
risks of a blocked catheter are considerably less.

The type of catheter to use immediately after prostatectomy is a matter of personal choice for the surgeon. Most
surgeons today prefer a self-retaining catheter with a Foley-
type balloon. The size of the balloon depends on the size of the
prostatic cavity left after prostatectomy. Provided no traction
is put on the catheter itself, a small balloon of about 5 ml is
often adequate. If, however, there is a large prostatic cavity
and no attempt has been made to obliterate this cavity at the

time of prostatectomy, then it is preferable to use a 20 ml balloon. On the other hand, the space occupied by the inflation channel for the balloon may, in the opinion of some surgeons, be better used to increase the lumen of the catheter, in which case a Harris or Nelaton type catheter is used without any self-retaining balloon. Fixation of this catheter to the penis can then be made with spirally fitting strapping[43]. It is unwise to use a stitch through the frenum as I have found on one occasion the patient had succeeded in pulling the catheter out and the stitch tore through the frenal artery requiring immediate return to the theater. It has also been suggested that the catheter could be anchored by a stitch through the abdominal wall onto a button. Organisms, however, found beneath such a button have been identical to the organisms found in the bladder. For this reason, it is suggested that this type of anchorage gives a further possible track for infection to enter. The pipe cleaner method advocated many years ago has two disadvantages: namely, poor access to the external meatus for toilet, and, secondly, a catheter can occasionally extrude between the external meatus and the pipe cleaners. My personal preference is for a Foley-type self-retaining catheter with a small 5 ml balloon.

The catheter is removed when the drainage is free of clots, usually on the second or third post-operative day, except when a transvesical prostatectomy has been performed, in which case the removal is probably about the fifth post-operative day. Before removal of the catheter, 50 ml of 1/5000 chlorhexidine digluconate is introduced into the bladder. The catheter is then removed, leaving the chlorhexidine in the bladder, to be passed with the first micturition after removal of the catheter. This has been found to reduce considerably the incidence of 'catheter fever'. The reason for this catheter fever would appear to be the first passage of urine when organisms can be found in profusion, despite the fact that the next passage of urine is sterile. It seems likely that the initial micturition clears some organisms contaminating the distal urethra, and the passage of the urine over the inflamed urethral mucosa probably increases the risk of absorption. If 50 ml of chlorhexidine is added to the urine initially passed, this risk is reduced considerably.

By these precautions of aseptic and antiseptic care in the operating theater, a closed drainage system post-operatively, with maintenance of meatal toilet, and the addition of 50 ml of 1/5000 chlorhexidine to the bladder just before removal of the catheter, the infection rate of post-operative prostatectomy has been reduced from somewhere in the region of 90% down to 7%[44].

Mortality and morbidity
When considering the mortality of prostatectomy by any route, it behoves us to recall the figures for prostatectomy 70 years ago, when Freyer[17] described his operation for total removal of the prostate gland. The word 'total' was in fact a misnomer as we have subsequently come to appreciate. The adenoma of the prostate, in fact, was enucleated from the compressed prostatic tissue which formed a false capsule. Freyer claimed that this was an adventitious layer of compressed tissue and did not contain prostatic glands. This erroneous assumption was probably due to the fact that most of his patients had longstanding urinary infection. Despite the type of anesthesia available at that time, the lack of antibiotics to deal with urinary infection, and the relatively poor endoscopic equipment to inspect the bladder and prostate pre-operatively, his mortality, he claimed, was only 5%. Even today, there are few series of open surgery for the prostate gland which can claim a mortality of less than 5%, when the surgeon has honestly accepted a true cross-section of all prostatic surgery with no geriatric limitations. However, it should be remembered that, in the days of Freyer, most patients had been on catheter drainage for some time, either *per urethram* or via a suprapubic cystostomy, and those with any cardio-respiratory limitations either succumbed during the period of catheter drainage, or were subsequently not accepted for open surgery.

O'Flynn[29] gave a review of the mortality for open prostatectomy as compared with transurethral surgery, which showed that the latter had an approximate mortality of only 1%. However, again one must remember that selection for transurethral surgery means on the whole a smaller gland with more fibrous reaction and less likelihood to bleed profusely.

The morbidity following prostatectomy can be summarized under (1) the effects of infection, (2) damage to adjacent structures such as the external sphincter of the urethra, resulting in incontinence, or the distal urethral mucosa, resulting in stricture, (3) the general systemic effects of surgery in the geriatric age group.

The work of Wilson Hey[22] in Manchester and Miller[40,41,42] et al. in Bristol has drawn attention to the serious post-operative effects of persistent urinary tract infection following prostatectomy. From the situation where infection was accepted in 90% of post-operative prostates, and surgeons tended to assume that the natural defence mechanisms of the body would deal with all of these infections, we have now come to realize that, far from dealing with these infections, there is a tendency for the organism to establish itself in a chronic inflammatory condition with the development of chronic lower urinary tract symptoms or upper urinary tract pyelonephritis with calculus formation. The significance of a small proteus colony count of 10 000 per ml even with relatively little tissue reaction in the form of a very low white cell count in the urine is now recognized as a potential precursor of persistent post-operative trouble, particularly if the organism is a proteus. Rigid drill in the management of the catheter and every possible attention to pre-operative, operative and post-operative asepsis and antisepsis has reduced the level of urinary tract infection to less than 7%.

The risks of post-operative incontinence are negligible provided the surgeon has orientated himself clearly with his landmarks of transurethral resection and has ensured at open operation that there is no damage to the mucosa below the lower border of the prostate gland itself.

Stricture of the urethra has been reduced to a minimum as a result first of reducing the size of the instrument used, secondly, ensuring adequate lubrication of the instrument, thirdly, the use of smaller post-operative catheters of non-irritant material and, finally, the condemnation of the old practice of prolonged pre-operative catheter drainage.

This leaves us with the final but unassessable problem of the effects of surgery in the geriatric age group. One must accept the fact that convalescence will be twice as slow and twice as long in the patient of 80 years of age when compared with the patient of 60. Furthermore, although we are well aware that the man of 60 will often volunteer the information that he is very much better two months after prostatectomy than he was pre-operatively, and has suffered no ill effects from the operation, nevertheless a similar assessment for the man of 80 years of age is not so often possible. Although we may be content with our figures for the mortality of the operation, it is very difficult to assess, at 80 years of age, whether the patient has recovered all his mental faculties completely at the end of three months convalescence. It is an almost unanswerable question for the relatives when they are asked "is grandfather quite as mentally alert as he was before the operation?". Particularly in this group of patients there is scope for an alternative form of treatment.

REFERENCES

1. Bartholinus, T. (1668). *Anatomy*, p. 377. Published by Nich, Culpepper and Cole
2. Paré, Ambroise (1691). *An Introduction to Chirurgery: the Anatomy of Man's Body.* Book 19, p. 445
3. Chopart, M. (1792). *Traite des Maladies des Voies Urinaires, (Vol. 2 des maladies de la vessie)*. Paris: L'Auteur
4. Desault, P. J. (1803). *Oeuvres Chirurgicales*, Retention d'urine par le gouflement de la prostate. Vol. 3, p. 220. (Paris: Mequignon)
5. Hunter, J. (1788). A Treatise on the Venereal Disease. Ed. 2
6. Home, E. (1811). Practical Observations on the Treatment of Diseases of the Prostate Gland, p. 118. (London: W. Balmor and Co.)
7. Guthrie, G. J. (1834). *The Anatomy and Disease of the Neck of the Bladder.* (London: Burgess and Hill)
8. Guthrie, G. J. (1834). On the Chronic Thickening of the Neck of the Bladder. *Lond. Med. Surg. J.*, 6, 321
9. Mercier, L. A. (1836). Recherches Anatomiques sur la Prostate des Veillards, *Bull. Soc. Anat. de Paris*, 3rd series, 2, 12
10. Civiale, J. (1823). *Nouvelles Considerations sur la Retention d'Urine*, p. 51. (Paris: L'Auteur, Bechet, Delauney)
11. Civiale, J. (1847). *Traite Practique sur les Maladies des Organes Genito-Urinaires.* (Paris: Bailliere)
12. Thompson, H. (1888). *Diseases of the Urinary Organs.* (London: Churchill)
13. Harrison, R. (1884). Treatment of Certain Cases of Prostatic Obstruction by a Section of the Gland, Proc. 8th Int. Med. Cong., Copenhagen. (Liverpool: Marples)
14. Gouley, J. W. S. (1885). Some points in the surgery of the hypertrophied prostate. *Trans. Amer. Surg. Ass.*, 3, 163
15. Goodfellow, G. (1904). Prostatectomy in general, especially by the perineal route, *J. Amer. Med. Ass.*, 43, 1448

16. McGill, A. F. (1889). The treatment of retention of urine from prostatic enlargement, *Brit. Med. J.*, *2*, 863

17. Freyer, P. J. (1901). Total extirpation of the prostate for radical cure of enlargement of that organ, *Brit. Med. J.*, *2*, 125

18. Thomson-Walker, J. W. (1904). The Prostate and Prostatectomy, *Brit. Med. J.*, *1*, 728

19. Harris, S. H. (1928). Prostatectomy with complete closure, *Med. J. Aust.*, *2*, 288

20. Kümmel, H. (1889). Die operative behandlung der urinretention bei prostatahypertrophie, *Verhandl. Deutsch. Gesellsch Chir.*, *18*, 148

21. Duval, P. (1906). Prostatectomie transvesicale avec suture de la vessie a l'uretre et reunion par premiere intention. *Bull. Soc. Chir.*, *32*, 651

22. Hey, W. H. (1945). Asepsis in prostatectomy, *Brit. J. Surg.*, *33*, 41

23. Millin, T. (1945). Retropubic Prostatectomy: a new extra-vesical technique, *Lancet*, *2*, 693

24. Hryntschak, T. (1955).Suprapubic Prostatectomy. (Thomas Springfield)

25. Mitchell, J. P. (1961). Reflections on the Indications for Prostatectomy, *Med. J. S. W.*, *76*, 85

26. Mitchell, J. P. (1972). The Principles of Transurethral Resection and Haemostasis (Bristol: John Wright)

27. McCarthy, J. F. (1923). A New Type Observation and Operating Cysto-urethroscope, *J. Urol.*, *10*, 519

28. Stern, M. (1926). Resection of Obstructions at the Vesical Orifice: New Instruments and a New Method, *J. Amer. Med. Ass.*, *87*, 1726

29. O'Flynn, J. D. (1967). Prostatectomy. A Review of 3083 Cases, *J. Irish Med Ass.*, *60*, 311

30. Mitchell, J. P. (1970). Transurethral resection, *Brit. Med. J.*, *3*, 241

31. Mitchell, J. P. (1955). Leg Stirrups for Cystoscopy, *Lancet*, *1*, 848

32. Miller, A., Mitchell, J. P. and Brown, N. J. (1969). The Bristol Bladder Tumour Registry, *Brit. J. Urol.*, *41*, Suppl. 1

33. Mitchell, J. P. (1958). A Simple Resectoscope, *Lancet*, *1*, 84

34. Mitchell, J. P. (1965). Resectoscope modifications, *Brit. J. Urol.*, *37*, 479

35. Hopkins, H. H. (1969). *New Optical Techniques in Medical Endoscopy*. Presented at 33rd Scientific Meeting of Biological Engineering Society at Middlesex Hospital, London (11 Jan.)

36. Alder, V. G., Gingell, J. C. and Mitchell, J. P. (1971). The Disinfection of cystoscopes by sub-atmospheric steam and steam and formaldehyde at 80 ° C. *Brit. Med. J.*, *3*, 677

37. Mitchell, J. P. and Lumb, G. N. (1966). *A Handbook of Surgical Diathermy*. (Bristol: Wright)

38. Swinney, J. and Hammersley, D. P. (1963). *A Handbook of Operative Urological Surgery*, p. 187. (Edinburgh and London: Livingstone)

39. Mitchell, J. P. (1952). A bladder Neck Spreader, *Lancet*, *1*, 193

40. Miller, A., Gillespie, W. A., Linton, K. B., Slade, N. and Mitchell, J. P. (1958). Post-operative infection in urology, *Lancet*, *2*, 608

41. Miller, A., Gillespie, W. A., Linton, K. B., Slade, N. and Mitchell, J. P. (1960). Catheter drainage and infection in acute retention of urine, *Lancet*, *1*, 310

42. Miller, A., Gillespie, W. A., Linton, K. B., Slade, N. and Mitchell, J. P. (1960). Prevention of urinary infection after prostatectomy, *Lancet*, *2*, 886

43. Mitchell, J. P. (1969). Urology for Nurses, 2nd Ed., p. 55. (Bristol: Wright)
44. Mitchell, J. P. and Gillespie, W. A. (1964). Bacteriological Complications from the Use of Urethral Instruments: Principles of Prevention. *J. Clin. Path.*, *17*, 492

4

Cryosurgical treatment for benign and malignant prostatic disease

N. Alan Green

Introduction

Destruction of prostatic tissue with low temperature was pioneered by Gonder and Soanes, Buffalo, New York[1], following its successful application in the neurosurgical treatment of Parkinson's disease by Cooper[2,3], and in cataract surgery by Krwawicz[4]. The freezing and subsequent thawing of the prostate induces necrosis, cryoprostatectomy being realized as cavitation takes place with separation of dead tissue. The refrigerant of choice is liquid nitrogen which, by virtue of its boiling point of $-196\,^{\circ}\mathrm{C}$, allows extreme temperature gradients, although nitrous oxide cooling to $-90\,^{\circ}\mathrm{C}$ has also been used[5].

APPARATUS

The original cryosurgical unit was designed by the Linde Division of the Union Carbide Corporation and is now produced by Frigitronics Incorporated, Connecticut, U.S.A.* This apparatus has been used by the author and will be described. Other units with some technical modifications achieve similar results, including that produced by Spembly Technical Products Limited.†

The apparatus consists of a cabinet on the front of which is a control panel of switches and dials. These activate the various electronic circuits, control the flow of liquid nitrogen and regulate and record temperature within the active portion of the cryosurgical probe. The liquid nitrogen container, feed

---

* Down Bros. and Phelps Ltd.,

† Spembly Ltd., Andover, Hampshire, England, Davis Keeler Ltd.

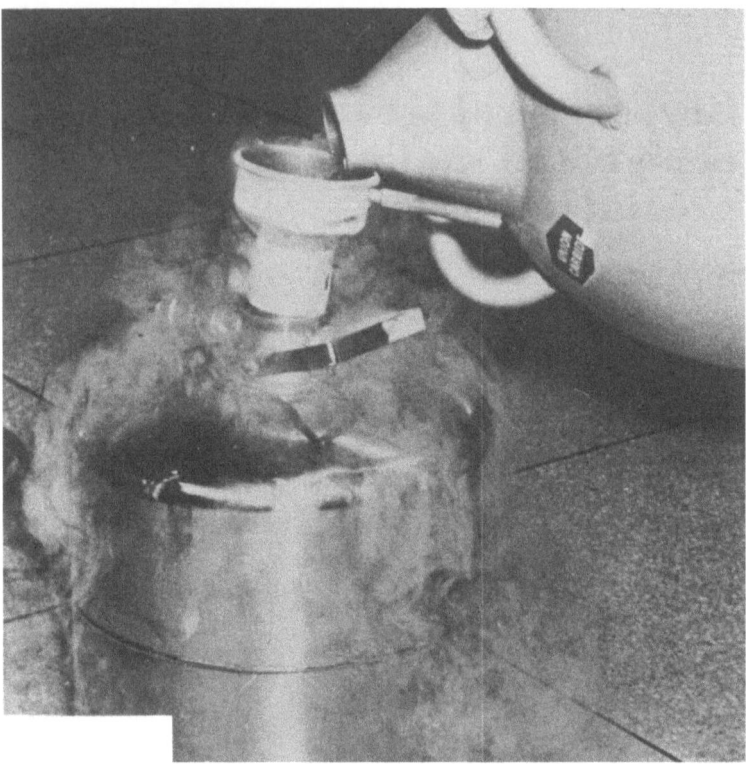

Figure 4.1   Pouring liquid nitrogen into Dewar container

line and cryosurgical probe are all vacuum-insulated except for the freezing segment of the probe through which heat transfer occurs, and unless a fault develops in this insulation only those areas near or in contact with this non-insulated segment will be subject to the cold trauma. The cryosurgical probe itself is 26 French in diameter and is shaped like a urethral sound. Liquid nitrogen is stored in large containers under low pressure conditions and is poured into the stainless steel Dewar container of 5 liter capacity. (Figure 4.1), and after being placed in position in the control cabinet is connected to the feed line and cryosurgical probe (Figure 4.2). Through a system of electronically controlled circuits the pressure of liquid nitrogen within the container can be raised to 28–30 lbs per square inch then allowed to flow from the container to the

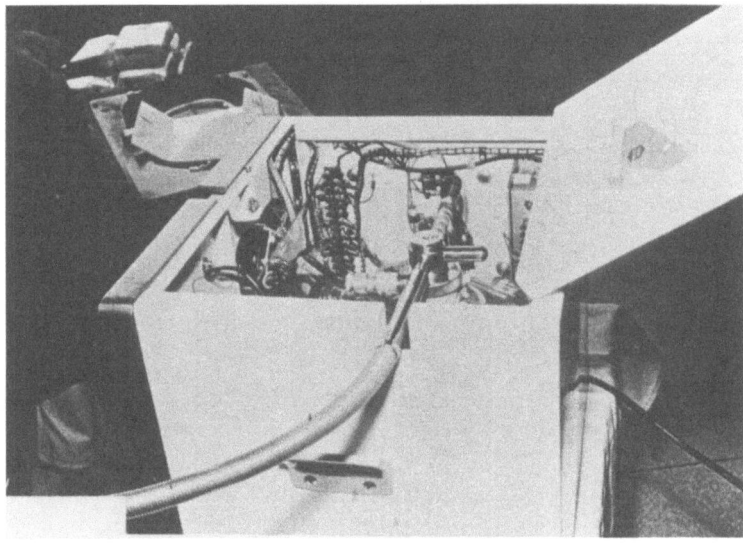

Figure 4.2   Cabinet and feed line attached to Dewar container

probe by activating the appropriate switches on the control panel (Figure 4.3).

Liquid nitrogen is thus fed through an inlet tube down to the probe tip where it undergoes gaseous transformation, the gas escaping along an outer tube in the feed line. The rate of escape determines the temperature of the non-insulated copper sleeve adjacent to the tip of the probe, and this can be controlled by adjustment of the appropriate knob on the control cabinet, usually to a temperature of $-160\,^{\circ}\text{C}$. A thermocouple embedded in the freezing zone passes back through the system to an automatic unit which controls the escape of gas thus maintaining the probe tip temperature at a pre-set level. The copper freezing zone also has a heating element controlled by a switch on the front of the cabinet. It is thus possible to warm the gland adjacent to the probe.

A selection of prostatic probes is available with a freezing zone varying from 1.5–4.5 cm in length (Figure 4.4). A reference knob placed on the under surface of the probe is situated 1.7 cm from the proximal end of the freezing zone. The external diameter of the probe is 0.86 cm (26 French),

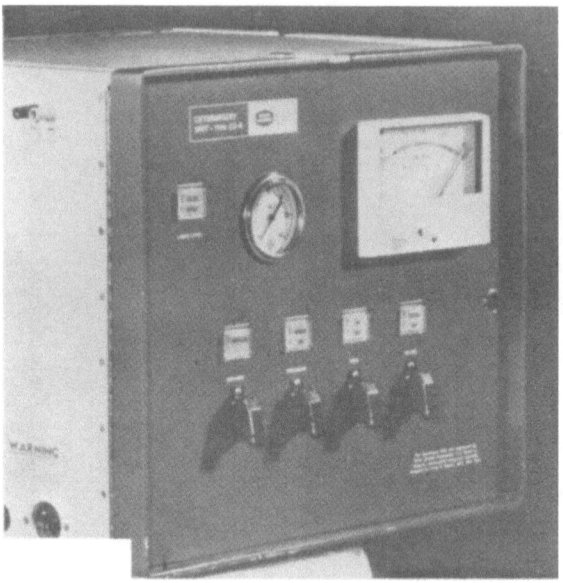

Figure 4.3   Front of control panel

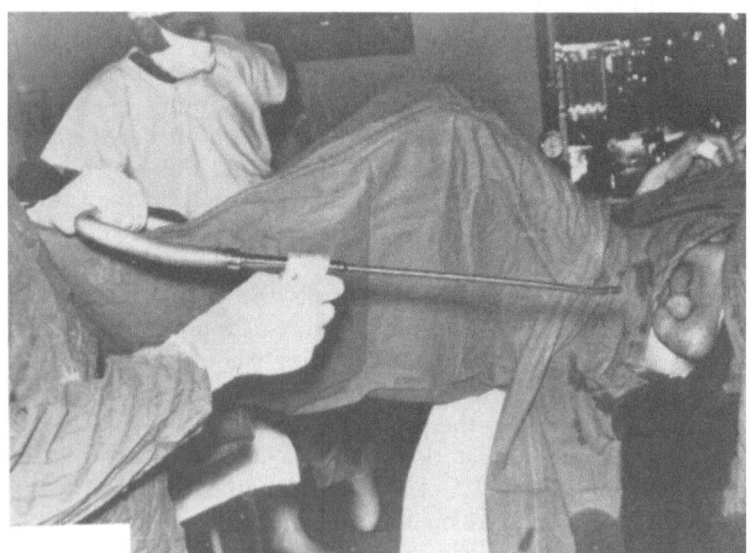

Figure 4.4   Cryosurgical probe prior to introduction

and has a minimal curve at its distal end to enable easy insertion and withdrawal along the urethra and to minimize freezing of the trigone of the bladder. An insulated tip, 1.4 cm in length, affords some protection against freezing contact with the bladder wall. Some idea of expansion of the ice ball formed during freezing can be seen by placing the probe in normal saline at body temperature which has an osmolality similar to that of human prostatic tissue and applying temperatures of $-160\,^{\circ}\mathrm{C}$ to the probe. Ice ball expansion occurs around the copper freezing zone and extends, to some extent, backward toward the reference knob and also proximally to the insulated tip (Figure 4.5).

After the required duration of freezing has been achieved the copper segment is re-warmed and the flow of liquid nitrogen into the probe is terminated. Re-heating of the probe does not cause complete thawing of the ice ball. A good account of the functional anatomy of the cryosurgical unit is given by Dow et al.[6].

TECHNIQUE
Patients can be subjected to cryosurgery using intra-urethral local anesthesia in the form of 4% lignocaine gel with Hibitane, under neurolept anesthesia or a very light general anesthetic.

Preliminary cystoscopy is followed by evacuation of all fluid from the bladder which is then distended with air using a bladder syringe to a capacity of 200–400 ml. This precaution is necessary to avoid contact of the bladder wall with the probe and in order to prevent any residual liquid contents from freezing. The well lubricated probe is then passed down the urethra and positioned so that the reference knob on the under surface of the probe can be sited at the apex of the prostate gland, confirmation of position being obtained by a finger introduced per rectum. With the handle of the probe slightly depressed to avoid any contact of the heat transfer area with the trigone of the bladder, the temperature of the probe is lowered to 0 °C in order to allow the probe to be fixed within the prostate gland, the lobes being massaged gently onto the probe by a finger introduced per rectum.

Reuter of Stuttgart recommends the use of a Trocar cystoscope introduced through the suprapubic area into the

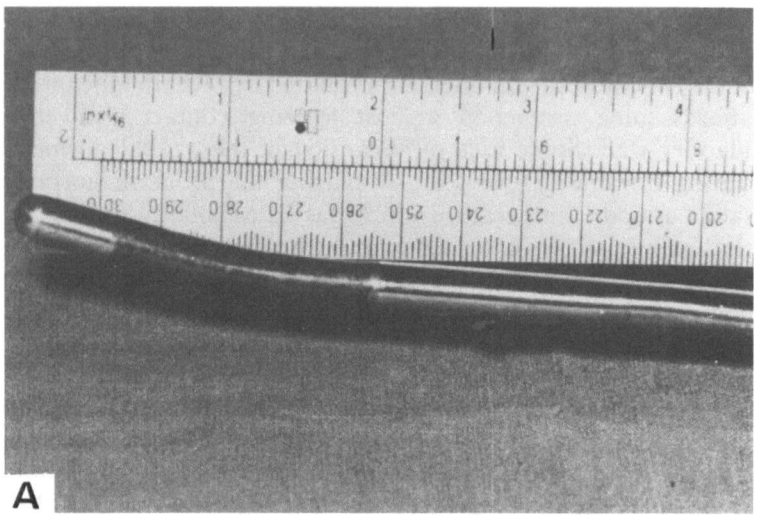

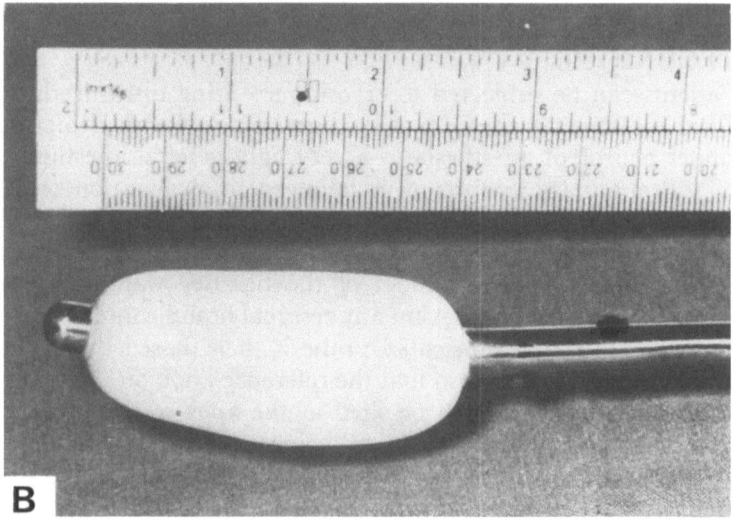

Figure 4.5   (A) Composite picture of freezing segment with expansion of ice ball in biological solution at (B) 3 min, (C) 6 min and (D) 12 min at − 160 °C

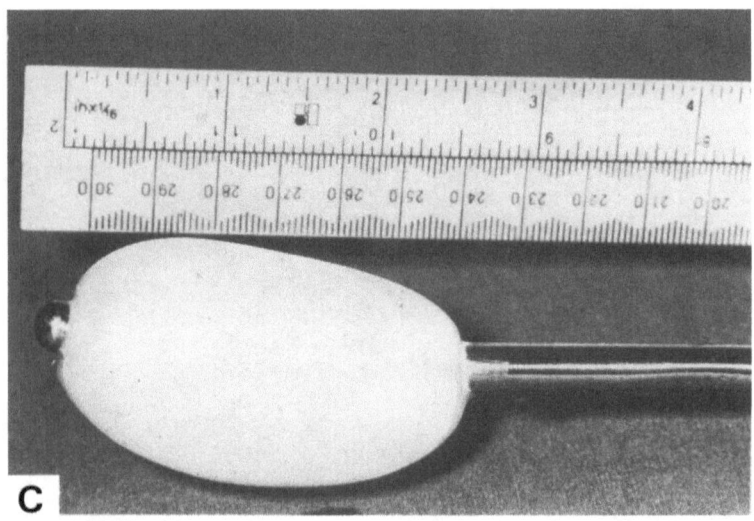

C

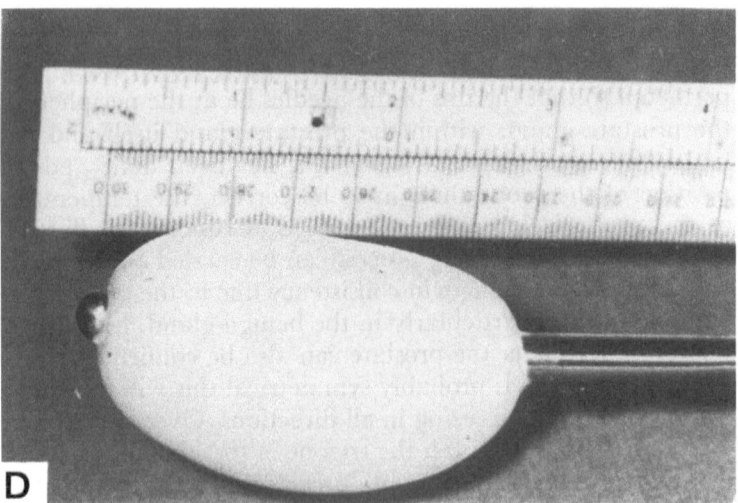

D

bladder in order to observe intra-vesical changes and to safe-
guard the ureteric orifices from damage due to the extension
of the 'freezing front'.

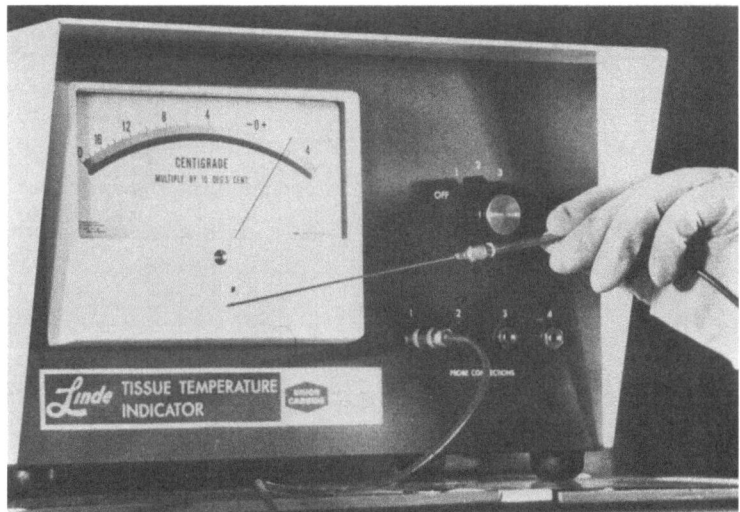

Figure 4.6   Thermocouple and tissue temperature indicator

Intraprostatic and rectal wall temperatures may be monitored by inserting thermocouples (Figure 4.6), through the
perineum so that the tips of the needles lie at the periphery of
the prostate gland, within the prostate gland itself and just
under the rectal mucosa. When this has been done and the
position of the probe thought to be correct, the temperature
of the probe is lowered to −160 °C. Crude, but effective,
evaluation of the freezing process can be carried out by rectal
palpation, when changes in consistency due to the growing ice
ball may be felt, particularly in the benign gland. Mobility of
the rectal wall over the prostate can also be confirmed. Since
ice ball expansion is probably symmetrical this will indicate a
rough extension of freezing in all directions. Over enthusiastic
rectal palpation may push the trigone of the bladder on to the
ice ball of the probe and a more precise control of the depth of
freezing can be provided by thermocouples. When the temperature reading at the thermocouple approaches that at which
cellular death occurs, freezing is stopped. A single thermocouple, providing accurate control in cryosurgical prostatectomy, has been developed by Fraser and his colleagues[7] with a
working temperature sensor of small dimensions including a

number of thermally and electrically insulated thermocouples evenly spaced along 10 mm of its length. The probe consists of a stainless steel hypodermic needle on which is mounted six copper constant thermocouples starting at a point 4 mm from the tip of the needle. The needle is mounted on the end of a plastic syringe which acts as a terminal support for the thermo-couple wires. In this way it is possible to provide information on the tissue temperature gradient continuously and at multiple points within and immediately outside the freezing zone, the surgeon being able to predict the precise position of the freezing front while it is still a safe distance from the periphery of the gland. On average, intraprostatic temperatures have been monitored at $-40\,^{\circ}\mathrm{C}$ to $-50\,^{\circ}\mathrm{C}$ and peripheral or capsular temperatures have varied in most series between $-6\,^{\circ}\mathrm{C}$ and $-20\,^{\circ}\mathrm{C}$. Certainly at $-15\,^{\circ}\mathrm{C}$ fewer complications appear to occur, and the experience of the author has suggested that a peripheral temperature of $-6\,^{\circ}\mathrm{C}$ is quite sufficient.

When the maximum or required cooling has been reached and the probe has been removed after re-heating, a plastic Foley catheter, size 18–22 French, is passed, using an inside introducer if necessary. Difficulty may be experienced in passing the catheter due to the rigidity of the prostatic urethra, and when prolonged periods of catheter drainage are envisaged the newer Silastic catheters are to be preferred. The length of freezing varies in most series from 4–16 minutes, the ice ball formed over the non-insulated portion of the probe gradually thaws, necrosis in the prostate gland being induced by what Soanes and Gonder[1] refer to as the 'freeze-thaw insult'.

PATHOLOGY

Changes following cryosurgery are essentially those of necrosis of varying degrees depending on the depth and duration of freezing, and the size, shape and vascularity of the prostate. These have been fully described by Gonder et al.[8]. The degree of necrosis is seen in Figure 4.7, as is widening of the bladder neck which is often one of the first radiological signs to occur. Immediately after thawing, swelling of the prostate gland and hemorrhagic infiltration occurs, persisting for 7–10 days (Figure 4.8). Necrosis of tissues commences with many ghost cells and breakdown in cellular membrane (Figure 4.9). The

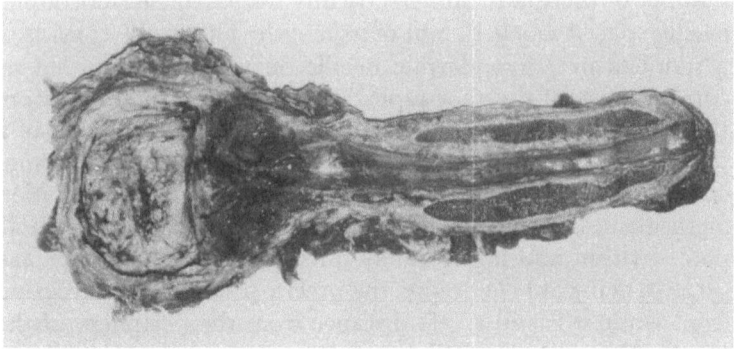

Figure 4.7 Post-mortem specimen indicating necrotic change in prostate. Note widening of bladder neck

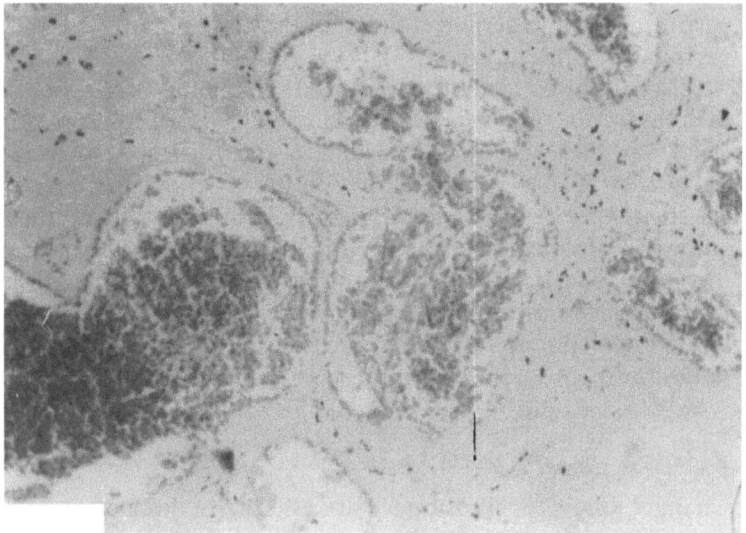

Figure 4.8 Slide showing hemorrhagic infiltration

presence of a peripheral inflammatory zone surrounding the necrotic area is evident as separation takes place and healing is achieved by re-epithelialization. Distinct fibro-blastic activity starts at 10 days after cryosurgery and glandular regeneration is seen after 3 or 4 weeks. At times haphazard regrowth occurs resembling neoplastic change. Squamous metaplasia of epi-

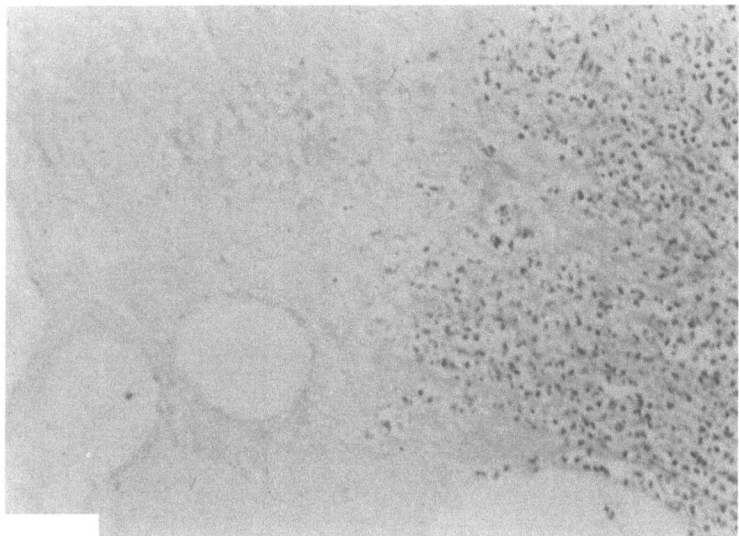

Figure 4.9   Slide showing necrosis and peripheral inflammatory reaction

thelial cells is quite marked, particularly at 3 months after the thermal injury. Dense fibrosis may occur in addition after a few months.

Histological studies of the human prostate some four years after cryosurgery have shown no evidence of malignancy occurring in a benign gland although occasional foci of squamous metaplasia are still seen.

RADIOLOGICAL CHANGES

Following cryosurgery the changes seen on radiography are those to be expected from a consideration of the pathological changes occurring in the gland, and depend on the degree of slough formation and its rate of separation. Clearly, this in turn is related to the size of the gland, the duration and depth of freezing and the effective vascularity in and around the prostate gland.

Little change is seen up to the 14th post-operative day on micturating cysto-urethrogram, except for slight widening of the bladder neck (Figure 4.10). There is a gradual widening of the prostatic cavity which increases up to a certain time, usually

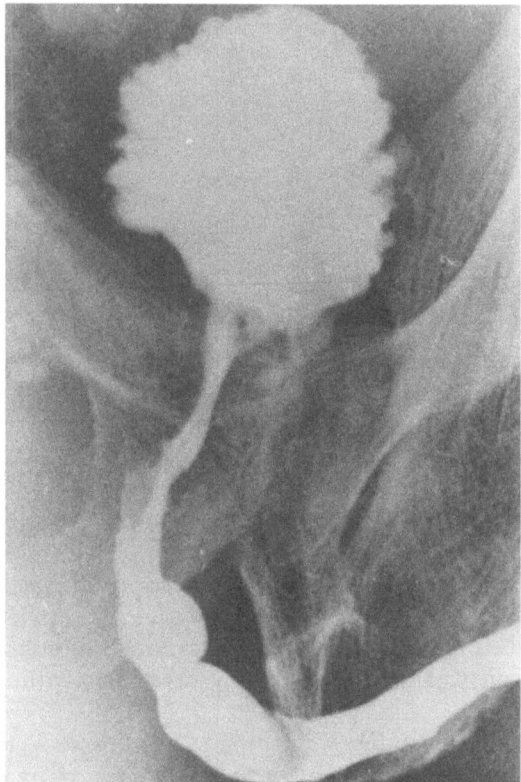

Figure 4.10   Radiograph showing widening of bladder neck

3 or 4 months (Figure 4.11). The calibre of this cavity may diminish slightly after 2 or 3 years, presumably due to regeneration of residual prostatic tissue. Smooth cavitation is seen in benign glands (Figure 4.12), after slough separation and occasionally irregular cavitation occurs in some cases of carcinoma, or asymmetrical enlargement of the prostate gland (Figure 4.13).

Rarely total opacification of the frozen prostate gland is seen at an early stage and may be indicative of massive slough separation at a later period (Figure 4.14). Of course, residual bits of slough may be seen at any stage before separation as filling defects in the prostatic cavity.

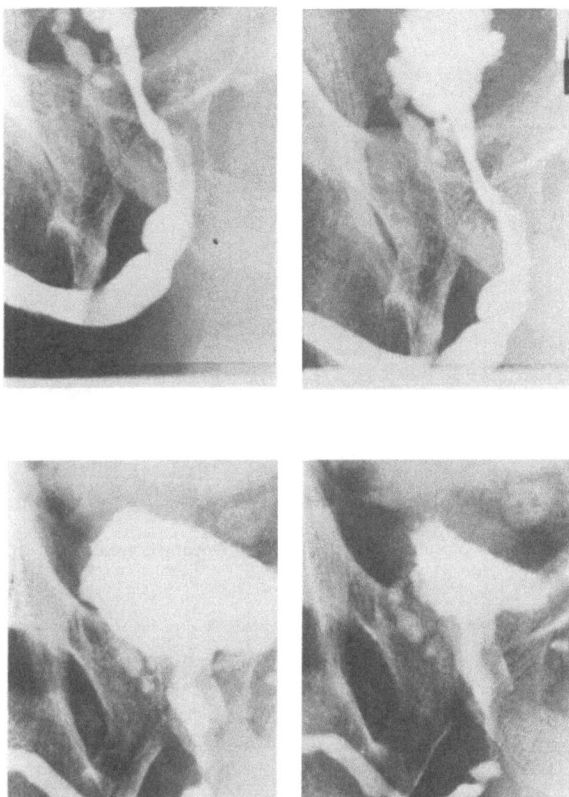

Figure 4.11   Micturating cysto-urethrogram taken at three weeks and three months after cryosurgery showing increase in cavitation

POST-OPERATIVE COURSE

Early mobilization is possible in most patients with a minimum of discomfort. Very little analgesia is required. Temporary penile edema is seen in about 5% of patients, often more marked about the 3rd or 4th day and settling quite quickly.

Very little immediate post-operative hemorrhage occurs, the total loss rarely exceeding 50 ml. More pronounced bleeding is usually due to attempts at removing the probe before adequate re-heating has taken place or to inadvertent freezing of the bladder wall. The urine remains tinged with blood for 12–24 hours and clears quite rapidly. Profuse bleeding is rarely

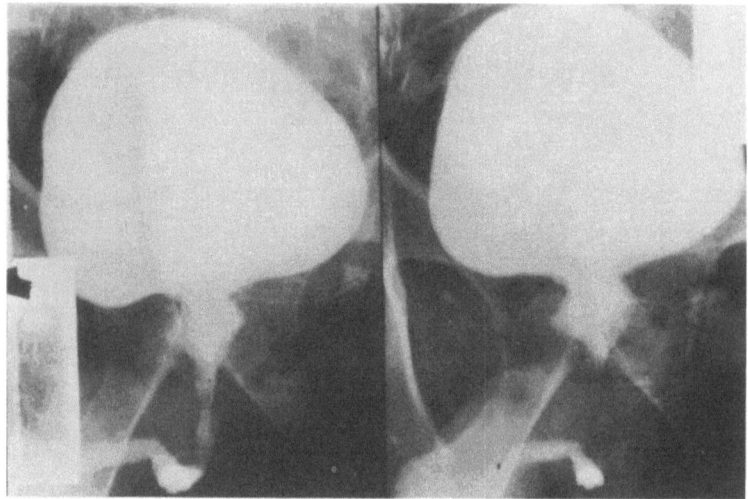

Figure 4.12   Smooth prostatic cavity 12 months following cryosurgery

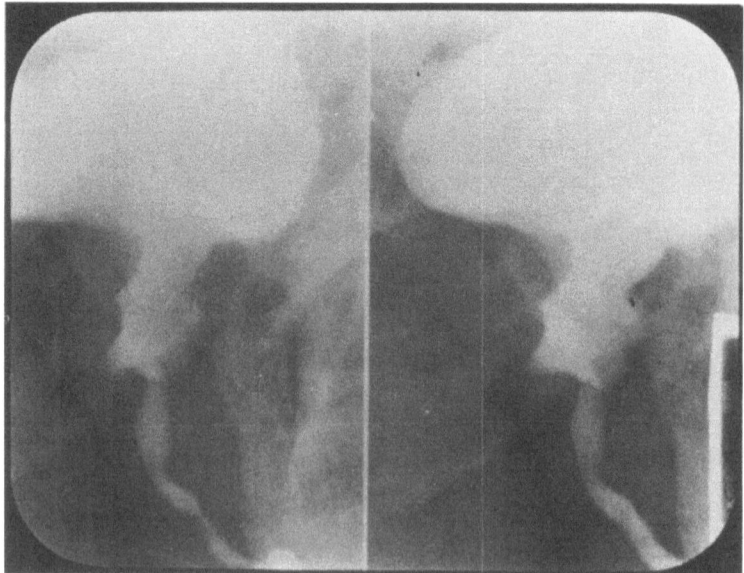

Figure 4.13   Irregular prostatic cavity in patient with carcinoma, six months post-cryosurgery

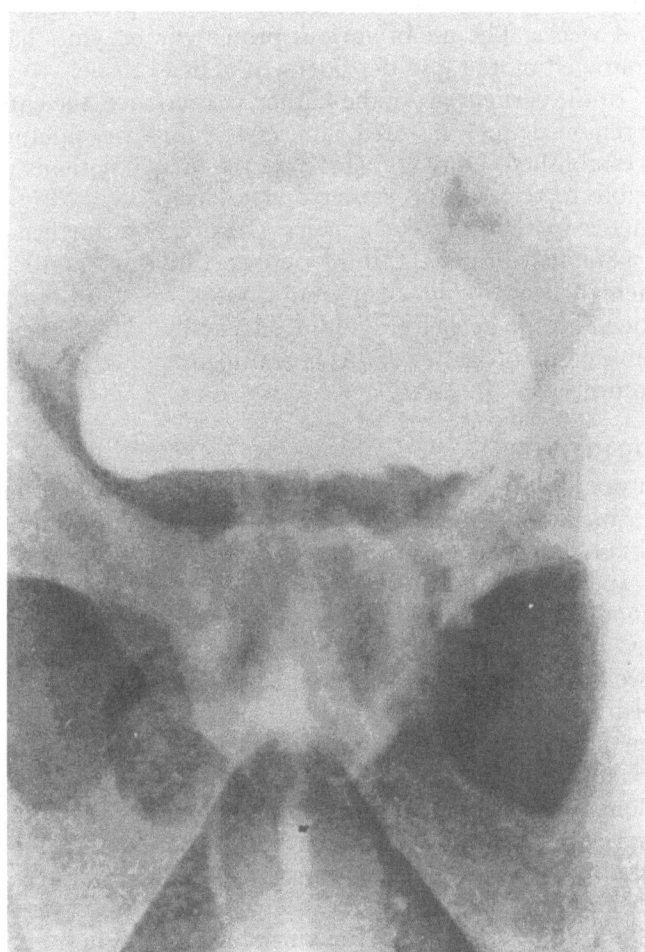

Figure 4.14   Total opacification of gland — early slough formation

seen[9] even with patients on anticoagulants or with blood dyscrasias. Secondary hemorrhage is uncommon and this is surprising in view of the known incidence of infective complications.

Clearly, the slow separation of slough is reflected in a more prolonged duration of catheter drainage than is needed in conventional prostatectomy. Most surgeons find a minimum of 7 days is necessary and in those patients presenting with large glands or urinary retention this may be prolonged up to 3 or 4 weeks. The use of various proteolytic enzymes has not encouraged more rapid debridement of dead tissue.

In the earlier part of the author's experience, the catheter was removed and reinserted, if necessary, until free micturition was established. Only in 6 (12%) of the first 50 patients was it possible to remove the catheter in under 8 days. 20% were catheter free during the second week and a further 28% (14 patients) during the third post-operative week. 40% (20 patients) needed three or more weeks of post-operative catheter drainage before voiding normally. This experience led to a policy of routine catheter drainage for 4 weeks following cryosurgery in all cases.

MORBIDITY

Post-operative complications may be related to over-enthusiastic or inadequate freezing, or to a faulty technique, and results probably improve with experience.

Infective complications are common but can be minimized by modifications in technique and appropriate chemotherapy. They are certainly lessened by leaving the patients with an indwelling catheter for a prolonged period of time. It would appear from personal experience that repeated catheterization when patients fail to void urine, or resection of obstructing necrotic tissue gives rise to septicemic episodes, ascending pyelonephritis or pyonephrosis in patients with dilated upper urinary tracts. Epididymitis has been reported but does not appear to be greater than with conventional prostatectomy. Over-enthusiastic freezing has led, on occasions, to peri-prostatic abscesses with pus tracking along fistulae in the groins. This complication is fortunately very rare. The size of separated necrotic tissue is usually small enough to pass in the urine almost unnoticed but obstruction by large sloughs does occur, occasionally necessitating re-admission for catheterization, particularly when the catheter is removed at an early date. Many surgeons find it necessary, with slow separation of slough, to perform a resectoscopic removal. Indeed, the combination of cryosurgery and resection has been advocated, but this seems an unnecessary elaboration of a technique which aims at a more conservative approach. Prolonged periods of catheter drainage is, to the author, a safer course to follow and patience is usually rewarded with success in voiding.

Incontinence of urine occurs, as in other forms of prostatectomy, and may be due to wrong positioning of the probe with consequent sphincter damage. At times loss of insulation results in an unexpected enlargement of the freezing zone and this may be a factor in the development of urinary leakage.

Some patients gain control of urine as all slough is separated and inevitably there is a hard core of patients who fail to control micturition whichever form of prostatectomy is employed. The overall incidence of this complication, once the technique is mastered, should be no higher than in other forms of prostatectomy, as is proved by personal experience.

Damage to the rectum has been reported occasionally with the production of a vesico-rectal fistula. Inadequate control of the freezing front of the ice ball is responsible for this complication.

Bladder wall damage occurs in patients with a small bladder capacity when it is difficult to distend the bladder away from the probe and from the ice ball. Damage to gut adjacent to the bladder wall may be seen and peritonitis is then a possibility. These complications can be reduced by the use of different sizes of probes, depending on the length of the prostatic urethra and the utilization of a more careful technique.

The incidence of strictures in the anterior and posterior urethra is low in most series and probably less than with endoscopic resection of the prostate gland.

Formation of bladder stones is surprisingly rare in spite of the fact that necrotic tissue has been reported in the bladder and prostatic cavity for periods up to 3 months.

Blood loss is certainly less than with conventional forms of prostatectomy and is nearly always less than 50 ml. Occasional patients do require bladder washouts for hemorrhage with clot formation. Secondary hemorrhage is a very rare complication.

INDICATIONS
Most surgeons who practise cryosurgery would accept that in a patient fit for major surgery, open or endoscopic prostatectomy is to be preferred. The cryosurgical technique is, there-

fore, most suited for a very unfit patient who is a severe respiratory cripple, or who has severe cardiac disability or even a recent cardiac infarct. The technique is ideal for patients with a limited life expectancy because of advanced malignancy in other sites, patients with a bleeding diathesis or on anti-coagulants.

The author has performed cryo-prostatectomy at the time of other major abdominal surgery, when retention of urine or severe prostatic symptoms are present. When prostatectomy is required for retention of urine occurring in patients soon after major surgery the technique offers some advantages to an open operation or prolonged resection of a large gland.

MORTALITY
It is difficult to assess the overall mortality from any reported series without an exact knowledge of the fitness of the patients in the series. Most series report a mortality of between 1 and 2%, but in some it is as high as 12% when cryosurgery has been used in the poor risk medical patient.

RESULTS IN CRYOSURGERY
The evaluation of the technique used on its own has been hampered in some series by incorporating the resection of prostatic slough in patients who failed to void at an early date. In most fully reported series with a 2 to 4 year follow up, radiographic, uro-dynamic and endoscopic studies have been performed.

There would appear to be a marked reduction in residual urine in well over 60% of patients following adequate cryo-surgery. Symptomatic improvement and measurable increase in flow rates is seen in at least two-thirds of patients but panendoscopic studies may show disappointing results. Kishev et al.[10] show the prostatic urethra encroached on, or deformed by residual prostatic tissue in two-thirds of the patients including those with good and poor results. In other words cryosurgical prostatectomy may never remove as much prostatic tissue as enucleation techniques or a good endoscopic resection.

MODIFICATIONS IN TECHNIQUES

With the knowledge of slow slough separation many surgeons are now prepared to leave a catheter indwelling for a month or more on the assumption that the necrotic tissue gradually separates and drains away.

In practice, simple rules have been evolved from personal experience.

1. Limitation of the duration of freeze to between 4 and 6 minutes for a gland between 25 and 40 g size and in glands over this size for up to 8 minutes using a temperature of −160 °C.

2. Early discharge of patients from hospital with an indwelling catheter if they were afebrile, mobile and without complications.

3. The use of chemotherapy during the period of catheter drainage.

4. Regular daily instillations of 1 in 5000 aqueous Hibitane solution.

5. To offer cryosurgery to all unfit patients who have a life expectancy longer than the intended period of catheter drainage, except for those who are severely mentally disturbed.

6. To re-admit most patients for twenty-four hours for a period of observation after catheter removal.

A review of a recent personal series of all types of prostatectomy and using the above guide-lines, showed that those patients undergoing cryosurgery and who were in a very unfit group had a shorter stay in hospital after surgery than those patients undergoing conventional forms of prostatectomy. Fifty-three patients undergoing retropubic prostatectomy stayed in hospital, on average for 10.3 days. The post-operative stay of 52 patients having an endoscopic resection was 8.6 days and 28 patients in a distinctly unfit category was further reduced to 4.5 days. A further re-admission was necessary for catheter removal, not exceeding 24 hours, in the majority of those undergoing cryosurgery.

CRYOSURGERY OF THE MALIGNANT PROSTATE

Cryosurgery may be used for the relief of urinary obstruction in the unfit patient with carcinoma of the prostate.

Total destruction of malignant cells is obviously difficult although techniques have been developed to separate the rectum from the prostate by surgery, freezing the prostate gland for 15 minutes or longer without fear of damage to the rectum. The application of a flat probe directly to the surface of the prostate through a perineal exposure has been described, but appears to have no real advantages, particularly if sequential cryotherapy proves to be beneficial in carcinoma[11].

Evaluation of cryosurgery as a sole means of treatment of carcinoma of the prostate is not possible at the present time. In addition to the local. destruction of malignant tissue, Soanes *et al.*[12] reported the demonstration of circulating antibodies to frozen prostatic tissue and made clinical observations on remission of metastatic lesions following cryosurgery and this suggested the possibility of an immunological effect of cryogenic destruction of prostatic tissue.

An initial immunological response was stimulated by freezing the prostate, and the tumor site was then re-frozen at a later date in an attempt to boost the production of prostatic tumor-specific antibodies by releasing antigens into the circulation which subsequently led to the destruction of previously rejected metastases. It would be unwise at this stage to elaborate further on the implications of this early work but new developments may be expected along these lines.

REFERENCES

1. Gonder, M. J., Soanes, W. A. and Shulman, S. (1966). Cryosurgical treatment of the prostate. *Investigative Urology*, *3*, 372
2. Cooper, I. S. and Lee, A. St. J. (1961). Cryothalamectomy—hypothermic congelation. *J. Amer. Geriatric Soc.*, *9*, 714
3. Cooper, I. S. (1962). Cryogenic surgery of the basal ganglia. *J. Amer. Med. Ass.*, *181*, 600
4. Krwawicz, T. (1961). Intracapsular extraction of intumescent cataract by application of low temperature. *Brit. J. Ophthalmology*, *45*, 279
5. Sesia, G., Ferrando, U. and Riggi, G. (1968). A new apparatus for use in the cryotherapy of prostatic destruction. *International Surgery*, *49*, 330
6. Dow, J. A. (1970). The functional anatomy of urologic cryosurgical unit and its relation to the technique complications and results of cryosurgery of the prostate. *J. Urol.*, *104*, 575
7. Fraser, J. (1972). Personal communication
8. Gonder, M. J., Soanes, W. A. and Smith, V. (1965). Chemical and morphological changes in the prostate following extreme cooling. *Annals N.Y. Acad. Sci.*, *125*, 716

9. Green, N. A. (1970). Cryosurgery of the prostate gland in the unfit subject. *Brit. J. Urol.*, *42*, 10

10. Kishev, S. V., Coughlin, J. D. and Dow, J. A. (1970). Late results following cryosurgery of the prostate. *J. Urol.*, *104*, 893

11. Flocks, R. H., Nelson, C. M. K. and Boatman, D. L. (1972). Perineal cryosurgery in prostatic carcinoma. *J. Urol.*, *108*, 933

12. Soanes, W. A., Ablin, R. J. and Gonder, M. J. (1970). Remission of metastatic lesions following cryosurgery in prostatic cancer; immunologic consideration. *J. Urol.*, *104*, 154

5

Conservative treatment of cancer of the prostate

G. D. Chisholm

Introduction

In many parts of the world conservative or non-operative treatment of carcinoma of the prostate is the standard form of therapy and surgical excision of the tumor occurs either incidentally with a routine prostatectomy or definitively for malignant obstruction. Conservative treatment has now assumed such a diversity of methods that this can only mean there is little agreement as to the optimal treatment. A host of questions have yet to be answered although some answers are slowly emerging and must now be recommended for clinical practice. Further controlled studies with adequate follow-up are still required to establish the place of surgery in relation to conservative treatment and to determine the exact form of this treatment.

Tumor staging

Any discussion of treatment and, in particular, comparison of data from several centers is restricted because of differing criteria for tumor staging. Recent progress in establishing a system acceptable to all urologists has yet to be consolidated but until this occurs the comparison of different treatments will remain unreliable and clinical impression will override fact. The two main staging systems in use for prostatic cancer are the UICC (Table 5.1) and the American (Table 5.2) and a comparison of these is given in Figure 5.1. Although there are proposed modifications to the UICC classification that will include still further subdivisions, it is hoped that this system will become more generally acceptable for there can be no substitute for the maximum of descriptive data from each patient.

Table 5.1 STAGING IN CARCINOMA OF THE PROSTATE AS RECOM
MENDED BY UNION INTERNATIONALE CONTRE LE CANCRUM (UICC)
IN 1967 (See also Appendix at the end of this chapter).

T   Primary tumor

TX   Incidental findings of carcinoma in operative specimen

TO   No evidence of primary tumor

T1   Tumor occupying less than one half of the prostate and surrounded by palpably
normal gland

T2   Tumor occupying one half or more of the prostate but not producing enlargement or deformity of the gland

T3   Tumor confined to the prostate but producing enlargement or deformity of the
gland

T4   Tumor extending beyond the prostate

N   Regional lymph nodes

NX   When it is impossible to assess the regional nodes, the symbol NX will be used,
permitting eventual addition of histological information, thus: NX − or NX +

NO   No deformity of the regional nodes on lymphography

N1   Regional nodes deformed on lymphography

N2   Fixed palpable abdominal nodes

M   Distant metastases

MO   No evidence of distant metastases

M1   Distant metastases present
   M1a   Bone metastases only
   M1b   Other metastases with or without bone metastases

Note: The determination of extent of disease should be based on clinical examination,
radiography and endoscopy.
The diagnosis must be confirmed by either:
(a)   microscopy (either by cytological or histological examination), or
(b)   combined radiography and biochemical tests (providing the serum acid
phosphatase is raised on two different occasions).
The regional lymph nodes are the intra-abdominal subdiaphragmatic nodes.

Tumor staging must begin with a tissue diagnosis and
when possible, should include serum acid phosphatase, bone
marrow aspiration, bone biopsy, radio-isotope bone scan,
radiological bone survey and lymph node biopsy and/or
lymphangiogram. It is evident that precise information concerning the spread of the tumor is essential for a treatment
policy and can only be made from the acquisition and evaluation of these measurements.

Table 5.2 STAGING IN CARCINOMA OF PROSTATE: DATA ARE BASED ON CLINICAL AND LABORATORY INFORMATION. THIS SYSTEM IS USED IN THE V.A. CO-OPERATIVE STUDIES

1. (or A) Tumor confined to prostate and not palpable
Incidentally diagnosed. Normal serum acid phosphatase and bone survey

2. (or B) Tumor confined to prostate gland but palpable or rectal examination as a nodule. Normal serum acid phosphatase and bone survey

3. (or C) Locally invasive either smaller than 6 cm in diameter (C_1) or larger than 6 cm (C_2)*. Normal serum acid phosphatase and bone survey

4. (or D) Distant metastases as judged by either biopsy, bone survey or elevated serum acid phosphatase. The prostate may vary from either normal (i.e. occult tumor) to obvious periprostatic extension

*Carlton et al.[41]

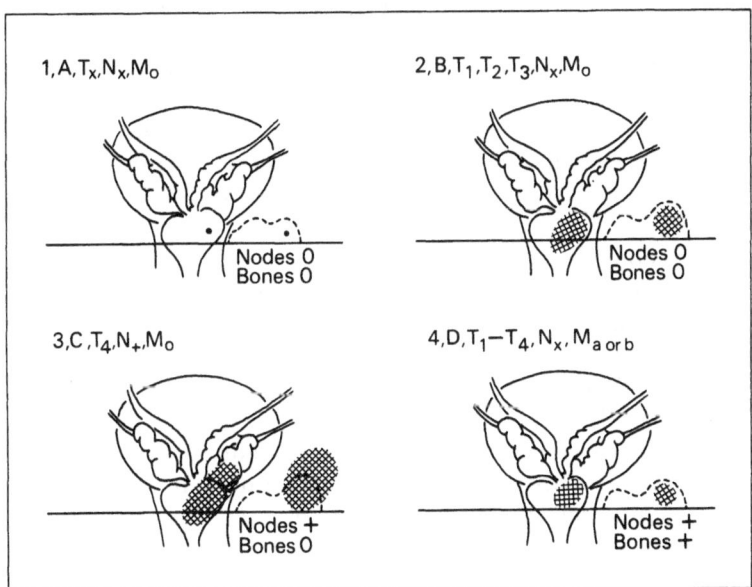

Figure 5.1 Comparison of staging methods for carcinoma of prostate. Adapted from Rubin[55]. By kind permission of the American Medical Association

Presentation

Carcinoma of the prostate is often asymptomatic until it has reached an advanced state so that there is some justification for using the terms clinical, latent and occult in relation to the presentation. Thus, the *clinical* tumor presents with symptoms of obstruction or pain and rectal examination reveals an obvious tumor; the *latent* tumor is that focus of tumor found at prostatectomy or autopsy with no other evidence of the disease; the *occult* tumor becomes manifest by its metastases for there is little or no local abnormality. While these terms may emphasize the variation in presentation they do not constitute a substitute for more accurate tumor staging. Indeed, in a series of random perineal prostatic biopsies in 688 virtually asymptomatic men (aged 50–69) Hudson[1] found localized carcinomata in 1 in 10. The detection rate for latent tumors undoubtedly increases where well-person screening is practiced and in some series as many as 2/3 of the tumors have been found as part of a routine examination. Whether or not the detection of these particular tumors has ultimately been to the advantage of the patient has yet to be demonstrated.

The average age at presentation in the series reported by Bumpus[2] was 65 with approximately 50% occurring between 60 and 70 years. More recent studies have shown that the mean age at presentation for all stages of the tumor is approximately 70 years. The tumor is rare under the age of 50, becomes increasingly frequent with age but after the age of 80 clinical cases become less common and latent cases are more common so that most men over 90 have these lesions.

The most common symptoms associated with carcinoma of the prostate are either obstructive (65%) or pain (25%) in the back, thighs or perineum. Approximately 10% of patients present with either hematuria or general debility. Bony symptoms rarely correlate with the extent of the disease as measured by either radiological or scanning techniques and bony symptoms, without evidence of metastases, should be regarded with suspicion unless screening tests including a biopsy are negative. Lymphatic spread is also difficult to assess without resorting to biopsy or lymphangiography; spread is mainly to the iliac and para-aortic nodes though Bumpus[2] reported that supra-clavicular nodes were involved in 11% and inguinal nodes in 18% of his series.

We have, therefore, a picture of a disease developing late in life, often asymptomatic and with a high incidence of spread that may not be evident by either clinical examination or routine radiology. Whereas 50 years ago there was little choice but to relieve any obstruction and await events, there is now a choice of treatments yet doubts have been raised as to the justification for giving treatment until symptoms (other than obstructive) are present. Such decisions can only be made on the basis of existing data for conclusions from relevant controlled clinical trials have not yet been reached.

Natural history
Some information concerning the natural history of untreated carcinoma of the prostate is available. In his review of 1000 cases Bumpus[2] reported that in 485 cases in which no treatment was given, the average survival from the first symptom to death was approximately 31 months and only 4 patients in this untreated group lived more than 3 years; when metastases were evident at the initial presentation, 2/3 of these patients died within 9 months. In a group of 125 patients in whom cystostomy was carried out for outflow tract obstruction the average survival was 57 months and this represented the best 'treatment' group. A collected series of 795 untreated patients formed the control group against which Nesbit and Baum[3] compared the early experience with hormone therapy. The 5 year survival rate with no metastases at the time of admission was 10% and 6% if metastases were present.

Table 5.3 LIFE EXPECTANCY IN MALES

U.S. male percentage survival*				U.K. male average life expectancy†	
Age	5 yrs	10 yrs	15 yrs	Age	Years
60	87	70	51	60	15.1
65	80	59	38	65	12.0
70	74	48	25	70	9.3
75	65	33		75	7.2
80	51			80	5.4

* Quoted by Grayhack and Kropp[51] from Vital Statistics of the U.S. 1963
† From Annual Abstracts of Statistics 1972. H.M.S.O., London

In assessing the natural history of untreated disease it is essential to give consideration to life expectancy tables (Table 5.3).

Endocrine therapy

Prior to the advent of hormone therapy, the treatment for carcinoma of the prostate aimed only to relieve urinary obstruction and pain. Direct radiation therapy was attempted but abandoned (see later). In 1941, Huggins published the first of a series of articles describing the rationale for treatment of prostatic cancer by endocrine manipulation[4]. Later, he wrote "The evidence for the facts which represent the premises was based entirely in the laboratory"[5]. In 1935 it had been observed that adult prostatic epithelium had a high acid phosphatase content and, in the following year, carcinomatous prostatic tissue as well as metastases were also found to be rich in acid phosphatase. To Huggins this indicated that malignancy represented an overgrowth of adult prostatic epithelium and since a reduction in androgens was known to produce atrophy of this epithelium, then castration or estrogen therapy should reduce the malignant activity.

The currently available evidence that a reduction in androgens affects prostatic growth has been examined in detail elsewhere[6] but the exact application of endocrine therapy in prostatic cancer continues to be debated. There is little doubt that castration or estrogen therapy can have a profound effect not only by shrinking the tumor but also by decreasing the serum acid phosphatase and controlling the metastases and anemia. In addition, the patient may have a striking subjective improvement. But not all patients respond equally, some may relapse and the treatment can produce its own morbidity and mortality.

The accumulation of acceptable clinical data from which to examine this response to treatment has been slow. The first major study, using data from 1818 cases, was by Nesbit and Baum[3] (Figures 5.2 and 5.3). The results with endocrine therapy were compared with a group of untreated patients collected between 1925–40. For those patients who were without metastases and treated by castration together with diethylstilbestrol (5 mg per day or less) there was a 5 year

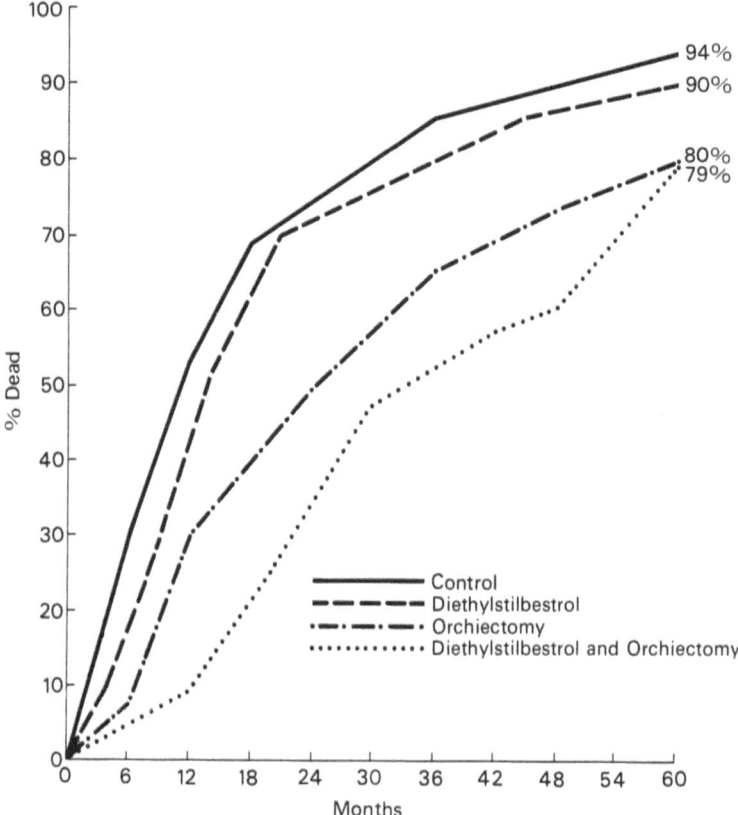

Figure 5.2   Five year survival of 263 patients with metastases at first admission. From Nesbit and Baum[3]. By kind permission of the American Medical Association

survival rate of 44% compared to the control of 10%. For those patients with metastases on first admission there was a 20% 5 year survival rate for both combined treatment and castration alone. While a large study such as this can easily be criticized for its retrospective character it became, for the following 20 years, the main reference point for the management of carcinoma of the prostate by endocrine therapy.

In 1960, Emmett *et al.*[7] reviewed their experience with endocrine treatment in 1101 patients but unfortunately the method of selection for each treatment group was not discussed. Their results showed that for those patients who

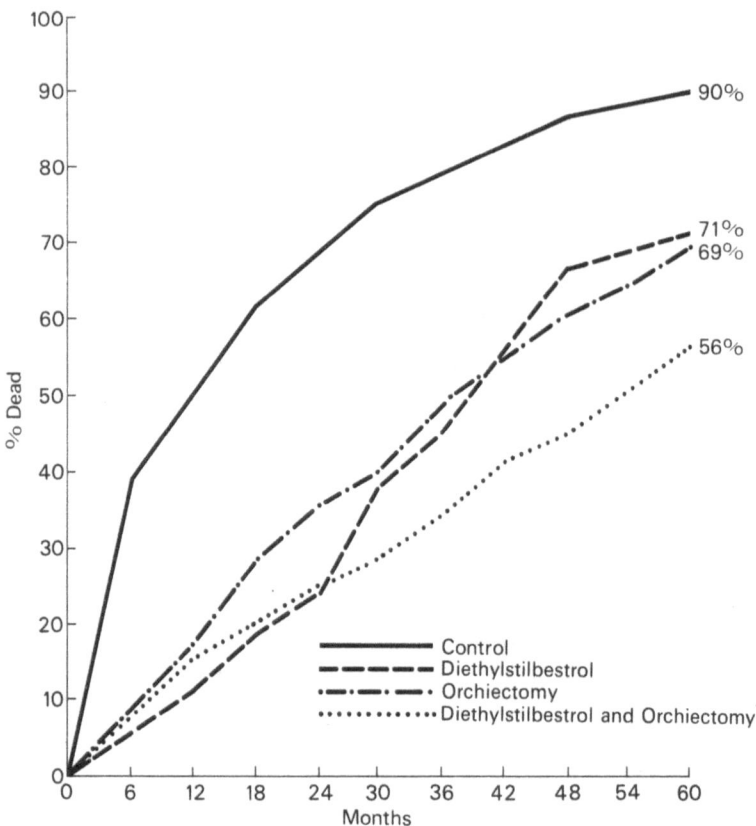

Figure 5.3   Five year survival of 324 patients without metastases at first admission. From Nesbit and Baum[3]. By kind permission of the American Medical Association

presented without metastases there was a 5 year survival rate of 56.8% for the orchíectomy group compared to 32.8% for the estrogen treated group. For those patients presenting with metastases the estrogen treated group fared slightly better (18.5%) compared to the orchiectomy group (13.5%). The 5 year survival in a group of patients that did not receive endocrine therapy was 15.4%. It was concluded that survival for patients without metastases was significantly increased by early orchiectomy rather than stilbestrol. Since the survival rates among patients who had metastases were so poor it seemed unwise to delay endocrine treatment until metastases appeared.

Where the tumor appears to be completely localized the attraction of a radical (curative) excision persists but the usual age of the patient at presentation and the doubts about the accuracy of staging have dulled this attraction for most urologists. Even more confusing, proponents of radical surgery have often included a bilateral orchiectomy as part of the operation. Thus, although endocrine control continues as the most commonly used treatment, albeit with a variety of treatment regimes and varying degrees of success, it is readily recognized as palliative.

A major problem in the use of endocrine therapy has been the unpredictable character of the disease. Franks[8] has emphasized that there are two types of prostatic cancer, one which behaves as an active carcinoma and eventually kills the patient and one other which is an incidental finding at autopsy. Histologically these appear to be identical but their biological behavior is clearly very different. There is also an important biological variation amongst the active tumors for there is a proportion, 10-20%, that show no objective response to endocrine therapy (see Chapter 1).

When Huggins[5] reviewed his early results with endocrine therapy it appeared that failure was more likely with an undifferentiated carcinoma. Subsequent studies of tumor grade and survival have been inconsistent: whereas Franks et al.[9] found no correlation, Schirmer et al.[10] have given strong support to the view that the grade of the tumor was an important factor in determining the incidence of metastases and the prognosis. It has been suggested that the grade of metastatic lesions may provide a more reliable prognostic index than the grade of the primary tumor[11].

Detailed histologic and biochemic studies have characterized normal, hyperplastic and malignant prostatic tissue (Table 5.4: from Grayhack and Wendel[6]) but, as yet, the features that indicate either persistence of normal endocrine responsiveness or lack of responsiveness have yet to be identified.

The choice between estrogens or castration either alone or in combination has been based largely on the study by Nesbit and Baum[3] where the results suggested the use of estrogen therapy in the absence of metastases and either combined

Table 5.4   COMPARISON OF CHEMICAL CHARACTERISTICS OF CAR-
CINOMA WITH NORMAL PROSTATE AND BENIGN PROSTATIC HYPER-
TROPHY. (FROM GRAYHACK AND WENDEL[6])

Characteristic	Normal prostate benign hypertrophy	Carcinoma
Acid phosphatase		Decrease (Q) Variable cellular reaction within and between tumor (H)
Acid phosphatase isozymes		? unique molecular form
Lactic dehydrogenase	No definite difference (Q)	
LDH isozymes		Increase LDH_4 and LDH_5
Aminopeptidase	Strongly reactive but may be absent (H)	Usually absent, not always (H)
β-Glucuronidase		? increase (H)
Esterases	No definite difference (H)	
Citric acid	High concentration BPH (Q)	Markedly reduced (Q)
Total organic acids malic acid, aconitic acid		Decreased (Q)
Pyruvic acid		Decreased (Q)
Lactic acid		Increased (Q:
Mucins	Neutral mucins (H)	Sulfated sialic acid containing mucins (H)
Copper	No definite difference	
Zinc	Marked increase compared with normal in BPH (Q & H)	Marked decrease (Q & H)
Magnesium	Marked increase compared with normal in BPH (Q & H)	Marked decrease (Q) Not demonstrable (H)

(Q) indicates quantitative data
(H) indicates histological observation

treatment or castration alone when metastases were present.
The hazards of giving estrogens in the presence of severe cardio-

vascular disease, the need for a rapid response and the possible futility of prescribing for a patient who may not take the tablets regularly are all indications for preferring orchiectomy and some clinicians believe this to be the most reliable initial treatment.

Others prefer to reserve castration for the patient who has relapsed after estrogen therapy. In this instance the suppression of testicular androgenic function 'escapes' control as judged by a rise in serum acid phosphatase and extension of bony metastases and subjective deterioration; orchiectomy may produce a useful though short-lived remission. While subcapsular orchiectomy may be more acceptable esthetically, it is possible to leave some androgen producing tissue so that a total epididymo-orchiectomy is to be preferred. Failure to respond to either estrogens or orchiectomy has led to the use of other measures to reduce the endocrine stimulus to the prostate, such as adrenalectomy and hypophysectomy (Chapter 6). Other measures such as radiotherapy or chemotherapy have been subjected to renewed interest.

Which drug?

ESTROGENS
The estrogens usually used to suppress androgen function have been either stilbestrol or diethylstilbestrol (DES). Natural estrogens such as ethinyl estradiol are more expensive and less active. No estrogenic substance has been demonstrated to produce a more complete or lasting suppression of pituitary activity in man or more adequate suppression of prostatic tumor cell growth than synthetic stilbestrol. Other drugs have been recommended but there is little objective evidence from which a choice can be made. When a patient has relapsed while on one estrogen then neither a change in dose nor a change to another estrogen has been shown to have any useful effect. It is, however, of considerable interest that a change to testosterone may produce appreciable palliation[12].

The synthetic estrogen chlorotrianisene (Tace) was introduced by Smith et al.[13]. Chemically similar to DES and hexestrol it was suggested that adrenal hyperplasia did not occur as with other estrogens and that side effects of dyspepsia, edema and gynecomastia were less. It has recently been shown that this substance is less effective in lowering serum testosterone levels than other estrogens. Thus, the current role of chlorotrianisene appears to be only as an alternative to stilbestrol should the patient be unable to tolerate this substance.

Estradiol phosphate (Estradurin) is an estrogen whose effect lasts for up to 4 weeks after one injection. Since it has only a weak inhibiting effect on gonadotrophins and yet has a satisfactory clinical response in patients it has been claimed that the action may be mainly by a direct effect on tumor cells[14] but there has been no evidence to support this hypothesis. As with chlorotrianisine, the main role of estradiol phosphate is as an alternative to stilbestrol especially when the patient cannot be relied upon to take the tablets and orchiectomy has been refused.

PROGESTOGENS

There have been several reports of favorable results with the use of progestogens in patients with carcinoma of the prostate[15]. Studies have been made with hydroxyprogesterone caproate (Delalutin), chlormadinone acetate (Chlormadinone) and cyproterone acetate (Depostat). Only a relatively few patients have been treated with each progesterone so that a useful comparison of survival rates with other estrogens cannot be made. It would appear advantageous to use a drug that has a significant effect on plasma testosterone and does not produce feminization but the mechanism of action in prostatic cancer is not known. In addition to the reduction of circulating androgen, chlormadinone acetate and cyproterone acetate may both suppress tumor growth through their peripheral antiandrogenic effect. The clinical improvement in patients with advanced malignancy has indicated the need for a more precise assessment of this group of antiandrogens and medroxyprogesterone (Provera) has been included in the V.A.C.U.R.G. Study III (see page 140 of this text).

CYTOTOXIC DRUGS

While both estrogens and progestogens may well exert some of their effect on the malignant cell by direct action there are two 'estrogen' compounds where cytotoxicity is believed to be the main effect.

Stilbestrol diphosphate (Honvan) is a phosphorylated synthetic estrogen formed by the substitution of a phosphate complex for the hydroxy grouping at each end of the stilbestrol molecule. It is water soluble (unlike stilbestrol) and almost inert estrogenically unless broken down by the enzyme phosphatase. This reaction results in the liberation of free stilbestrol from the phosphorylated compound and is believed to occur mainly in prostatic carcinomatous tissue, including metastases, where the concentrations of phosphatase are high and the requisite pH is present. Evidence to support these conclusions is incomplete: the results of biological assay have indicated that there is a concentration of stilbestrol in prostate tissue[16] but tracer studies have been less convincing[1]. Nevertheless, reports of the clinical response continue to show that stilbestrol diphosphate is well tolerated by the patient and has a particular use as a temporary form of treatment when a rapid response is required because of metastatic pain or urinary retention[18,19].

Estramustine phosphate (Estracyt) consists of a nor-nitrogen mustard which is linked to a phosphorylated estradiol. It has been developed for patients with more advanced disease where conventional therapy has failed and where the alternatives consist of hypophysectomy, adrenalectomy, radiotherapy or chemotherapy. The systemic cytotoxic and cytostatic drugs have been disappointing owing to their side-effects but estramustine acts by using the phosphorylated estradiol to carry the compound to the tumor tissue where enzymatic breakdown releases the nornitrogen mustard. The exact mode of action is not known but it appears to be more effective in depressing the activity of acid phosphatase and β-glucuronidase than estrogen alone[20].

Clinical experience with estramustine phosphate indicates that about 50% of patients experience good palliation for up to 3 years, especially the relief of pain[21]. Side effects of thrombophlebitis at the site of injection, marrow depression, nausea and vomiting have not been common and are not severe. It appears that this drug is valuable for palliation but should not replace conventional antiandrogenic treatment unless the patient presents with an advanced poorly differentiated tumor.

A variety of chemotherapeutic agents have been used for advanced carcinoma of the prostate including cyclophosphamide, mithramycin, triethylene thiophosphoramide (Thiotepa), actinomycin D and 5-fluorouracil. The results have been varied and, in general, not very encouraging[22]. The high incidence of side-effects, especially marrow depression, indicates that these agents must be modified before general clinical use is justified.

The dose of estrogen
In the original reports by Herbst[23] and Huggins and Hodges[4] patients with metastatic carcinoma responded to a dose of 1.0 mg diethylstilbestrol (DES) per day. Subsequently, other dosages were used in what was little more than a random attempt to find the optimum dose for the optimum clinical response. The majority of dose schedules were low and in the review by Nesbit and Baum[3] only those patients receiving the equivalent of 1–5 mg DES orally each day were included. Baker[52] found that as little as 0.25 mg DES intramuscularly per day would produce a remission. In 1954, Birke et al.[24] studied the urinary excretion of androgenic steroids (androsterone, etiocholanolone and total 17-ketosteroids) in relation to several dose levels and found the most rapid and effective response was with 30 mg stilbestrol per day for 5 days. With a dose of 10–15 mg stilbestrol per day the reduction in urinary androgenic steroids took 15–21 days and with 5 mg per day the effect was even slower. Thus, although it appeared that 30 mg DES was the optimum daily dose for suppressing pituitary trophic hormones there were no clinical observations to support this.

Fergusson[25,26] has recommended high dose levels (100 mg stilbestrol per day) and this has been widely used in the United Kingdom. Usually the dose is reduced to a maintenance level of 15 mg per day either within 2–3 months or when breast discomfort is evident. There has been little factual evidence that the high dose is better than a low dose regime except that Fergusson (1962) observed a better survival at 6 months with the high dose. The justification for these high doses has become increasingly uncertain from both clinical and biochemical observations. Recent studies have shown that the same reduction of plasma testosterone is achieved within about 7 days using doses of stilbestrol varying from 100 mg t.d.s. to 1 mg t.d.s. so that if the level of plasma testosterone is acceptable as an index of chemical castration then a higher dose regime is unnecessary[27]. It has also been shown that the optimum suppression of plasma testosterone throughout a 24 hour period is produced by a dose of 1 mg t.d.s.[28]. The measurement of plasma testosterone may also be a valuable index of the effectiveness of treatment and it has been recommended that this should be measured regularly in follow-up.

Bracci and Di Silveri[29] believe that the measurement of plasma testosterone has shown that estrogens do not completely inhibit either testicular or adrenal androgen production and that castration is the only procedure which effectively reduces the levels.

There remains the possibility that estrogens have a direct suppressive action on the prostate. Since the original work by Huggins and Hodges[4] it has been evident that estrogens act through the pituitary by suppressing Leydig cell androgen production. Farnsworth[30] has now produced evidence of a direct and suppressive effect of estrogens on the prostatic metabolism of testosterone *in vitro*. Possible mechanisms for this include competition for active centers on the androgen-metabolizing enzymes, or depletion of co-factors required for androgen metabolism. Since both estrogen and androgen cytoplasmic receptors have now been demonstrated in the prostate it may be that androgen metabolism is normally regulated by estrogens[31]. The significance of these observations in relation to the therapeutic dose of estrogen and to prostatic growth and function has yet to be established.

Radiotherapy
A variety of irradiation treatments have been used and these will be considered in respect of their route of administration:

LOCAL IMPLANTATION
Radium treatment for carcinoma of the prostate was introduced at the Mayo Clinic in 1915[2]. At first, it was placed in the rectum directly over the prostate but the resulting proctitis prevented adequate dosage. Later, the radium was given by

direct implantation of needles via the perineum and a per-urethral method was also tried but the poor results with all these methods eventually led to their abandonment[32].

In 1959 Flocks reported his experience with interstitial irradiation using radioactive gold (^{198}Au). This was used either alone or as an adjunct to surgical treatment at the time of prostatectomy. The dose (up to a total dose of 100 millicuries) was injected into multiple sites and could be repeated at 2 monthly intervals to destroy residual tumor[33]. Flocks claimed significant improvement in the results with early lesions and also a decrease in the incidence of local recurrence following surgical removal of the tumor[34]. However, it is difficult to assess the true value of the procedure since most patients appear to have had several supplementary forms of treatment so that the influence of the radioactive gold alone remains uncertain.

Experience in other centers with this therapy alone has been discouraging[35]. A more recent report has indicated that a technique of retropubic implantation of ^{125}I seeds is both simple and safe but follow up is too short and the use of supplementary treatment will again make interpretation of the effect of radioactive iodine alone difficult[36].

EXTERNAL IRRADIATION

Subsequent to the earlier efforts with local irradiation to the prostate it was often stated that carcinoma of the prostate was radio-resistant and it was not until Del Regato[37] pointed out that slow growing tumors regress slowly under irradiation just as rapidly growing tumors regress rapidly that the myth of radio-resistance began to disappear.

With the introduction of supervoltage irradiation it was possible to give a uniformly high dose to a precise area within the pelvis[38,39]. The dose to the prostate by current super-voltage methods is 7000–7500 rads in 7–8 weeks. When indicated, this may be combined with a dose of 5000 rads to the pelvic lymph nodes. The precision with which the dose may be delivered has minimized the complications to bladder and rectum but difficulty with micturition (30%), diarrhea (30%), rectal bleeding (5%) and incontinence (2%) may occur; potency has been maintained in 70% of patients[40].

Interpretation of reported results is handicapped by the high proportion of patients also treated with hormone therapy and by the difficulty in obtaining reliable staging of the disease. In an attempt to resolve the uncertainty of tumor staging Carlton et al.[41] have recommended retropubic exploration and pelvic node biopsy; in their experience 30% of clinical Stage C lesions were found to be Stage D at exploration. In that study, the radiotherapist implanted radioactive gold seeds into the exposed tumor and gave supplementary external irradiation during the post-operative period. Although some patients have also received estrogens it does appear that this has not improved the results and Bagshaw[40] has reported the following survival figures for radiotherapy alone:

Stage B	5 year	75%
	10 year	48%
Stage C	5 year	48%
	10 year	27%

Similar 5 year survival rates have been obtained by Del Regato[42] and Shida[43].

SYSTEMIC RADIOACTIVE THERAPY

In the presence of widespread metastases, symptomatic and objective improvement has been reported with the use of radioactive phosphorus (^{32}P). The rationale for this treatment is based on the fact that the radioactive phosphorus is localized in active bone and therefore in the new bone associated with metastases; it accumulates less rapidly in slower dividing normal tissues. Two millicuries of ^{32}P are given intravenously every 5–7 days and treatment is stopped when the white cell count and platelets begin to fall. It has been claimed that the addition of testosterone increases the effectiveness of ^{32}P but there is little evidence for this[44]. By contrast, parathormone has been used to create, upon its withdrawal, a rebound effect that results in an increased deposition of radiophosphorus in bone and tumors; dramatic relief of severe pain has been reported[45]. An attempt at perfusing the prostate with radioactive phosphorus proved technically and therapeutically unsatisfactory[46].

Experience with radioactive phosphorus has shown that the main use is in those patients with advanced bony metastases that are painful but it is also in this situation that more recently introduced drugs such as Estracyt (p. 133) are as effective and more easily administered.

V.A.C.U.R.G.

In any discussion of the choice of conservative treatment for carcinoma of the prostate full reference must be made to the controlled therapeutic trials for this disease that are being carried out by the Veterans Administration Co-operative Urological Research Group (V.A.C.U.R.G.). Few studies have provoked more discussion and though much of the comment has been ill-informed some criticism has been justified. Nevertheless, they must be acknowledged as the only significant trials for carcinoma of the prostate to have been reported and the results have led to a reappraisal af 'standard' treatments as well as to further study of the metabolic effects of estrogen treatment[47].

V.A.C.U.R.G. was formed in 1960 in order to carry out prospective controlled clinical trials of the treatment of urological diseases. Since then there have been three consecutive studies of treatment for cancer of the prostate. In Study I 3793 patients were considered but 1479 (39%) were excluded for a variety of reasons[53]. The patients were staged according to the system described in Table 5.2 and the following treatments were allocated randomly: for Stages 1 and 2, radical prostatectomy and placebo or radical prostatectomy and 5.0 mg diethylstilbestrol (DES) per day; for Stages 3 and 4, either placebo or 5 mg DES daily or orchiectomy plus placebo or orchiectomy plus 5.0 mg DES daily. All results were assessed on the initial assigned treatment even though the clinician may have changed that treatment if he considered it necessary.

The results for Stages 1 and 2 showed that the supplementary estrogens not only failed to increase the length of survival but there was also a higher incidence of cardiovascular deaths in Stage 1. In Stage 3 there were fewer deaths in those not treated with estrogens and although the actuarial survival curves for each treatment in this stage appeared very similar the results in the non-estrogen treated groups were statistically significantly better than the estrogen treated groups. There were no such differences for Stage 4.

There have been several criticisms of this trial and these deserve some comment. Since 39% of the patients were excluded it would appear that the remainder formed a highly selected group. However, most of those excluded had either had previous treatment (688 patients) or a second malignant lesion (229 patients) so that more than 80% of newly diagnosed patients were eligible for the study. There appears to have been one group of 403 patients, whose exclusion, because of their poor clinical condition, would not find general acceptance and these account for about 10% of the total in the trial. The fact that a high proportion of patients had their assigned treatment changed has also caused adverse comment but this has been defended on the grounds that to prohibit such changes would have resulted in many more patients being excluded initially. Finally it has been suggested that the groups were not comparable especially since such details concerning age, cardiovascular and other disease were not in evidence. However, statistical tests have shown that randomization was successful in respect of these variables[54].

Because the cardiovascular hazard of estrogens was well emphasized the next trial (Study II) was planned to assess the efficacy of different DES dose levels. 561 patients were treated in the following groups: for Stages 1 and 2 radical prostatectomy was compared with placebo; for Stages 3 and 4 there were 4 treatment groups: placebo, 0.2 mg, 1.0 mg and 5.0 mg DES daily. In addition, more information concerning the cardiovascular status of the patient was obtained than for Study I. The follow up for Stages 1 and 2 is thought to be too short for comment on the value of radical prostatectomy for these patients, but estrogens are not recommended (Byar, 1973). In Stage 3 the best results were obtained with the placebo and there were more cardiovascular deaths with 5.0 mg DES than with other DES doses. In Stage 4, placebo was the worst treatment and 1.0 mg DES was just as effective as 5.0 mg with regard to cancer deaths and all causes of death.

The recommendations based on Study II suggest that Stage 3 and Stage 4 patients should not be treated until they develop either symptoms (pain), or metastases or raised serum acid phosphatases and then they should receive 1.0 mg DES daily. It is recognized that a longer follow-up in this study could result in some change to these recommendations.

The role of radical prostatectomy for early stage prostatic cancer is far from settled (see Debate which follows below). V.A.C.U.R.G. have studied a group of 148 elderly men with Stage 1 lesions and although only a 6 year follow-up is reported they have reached the tentative conclusion that radical prostatectomy is unjustified for this stage[49]. Indeed, it is suggested that the results reported for radical surgery may be due more to the biological potential of the latent tumor than to the surgery.

In the most recent V.A.C.U.R.G. trial, Study III, the treatments for Stages 1 and 2 are the same as in Study II, but in Stages 3 and 4 there are three groups: Premarin (conjugated equine estrogens), Provera (medroxyprogesterone) and 1.0 mg DES are to be compared.

The fact that these trials have some limitations must not detract from the principle that future progress in the management of these patients depends on large scale controlled prospective trials.

Debate

It is frequently stated that a radical excision of the prostate for Stages 1 and 2 tumors is the only curative form of treatment for these patients and the comparison is made with some other early cancers where complete surgical removal results in 'cure' of the disease. Few would deny the effectiveness of this approach for some tumors yet a considerable debate exists as to whether or not the patient with early carcinoma of the prostate is best served by this approach. In most series of cancer of the prostate the mean age is about 70 years so that the life expectancy of these men is limited and they may have or are liable to have other diseases that may be fatal. Thus, a major surgical procedure in this age group becomes questionable unless the results are significantly better than other methods; in practice, radical excisions are restricted to patients under 70 in most series.

It is also questionable whether the early stage tumor can be compared with other prostatic tumors: it appears to be a different form of the disease being more resistant to radiotherapy and even hormone independent. Indeed, there is little evidence that these lesions progress to symptomatic metastatic cancer while latent cancers occur quite frequently in races where the (clinical) incidence is low. Those who have favored radical surgery have never doubted the validity of their arguments and they have never carried out a randomized clinical trial. In the V.A.C.U.R.G. Studies II and III, radical prostatectomy plus placebo is being compared to placebo alone in patients with Stage 1 and 2 tumors but although it is too early to draw conclusions, no differences in the two groups have yet been observed[49]. Until the long term survival from trials such as these become available, a comparison can only be made between series of patients treated either conservatively or radically where adequate follow-up data are available.

The incidence of death from Stage 1 cancer of the prostate, not treated by radical surgery, is very low and in a collected series (where the length of follow-up was variable) the incidence was approximately 2%. Thus, a non-surgical conservative approach to these patients appears justified though whether or not this is true for the younger patient with a more advanced grade of tumor requires further consideration.

Patients with Stage 2 lesions, a localized nodule, would therefore appear more suited for surgical treatment. However, Barnes and Ninan[50] have shown that the 10 and 15 year survivals for Stages A (or 1) and B (or 2) were similar in their series:

	10 year	15 year
Stage A	(30/58) 52%	(15/50) 30%
Stage B	(47/78) 60%	(21/58) 36%

Barnes and Ninan concluded that both Stages may be classed as 'early cancer' and their gross survival rates for these patients are 57% at 10 years and 33% at 15 years. 75% of the 15 year survivors were in good health though only 21% were without evidence of cancer.

The data for long-term survival after radical surgery are presented in Chapter 6 but it is reasonable to emphasize that although there may be a higher proportion of patients that are tumor free at 15 years the differences in survival rates are insignificant while that elusive factor in medicine, the quality of life, has not been quantified for either form of therapy.

APPENDIX

Modification of UICC classification of Carcinoma of the Prostate as recommended by British sub-committee 1974.

The diagnosis must be confirmed by histology obtained from the primary tumor or metastases *or* by needle aspiration of the primary tumor or metastases *or* by combined radiography and biochemical tests.

The determination of the extent of the disease is based on clinical examination, radiography, endoscopy and biochemical tests.

The regional lymph nodes are the pelvic nodes below the bifurcation of the common iliac arteries.

In addition to the TNM categories, P categories indicating the histological extent of disease within the prostate gland and G categories indicating the grade of the tumor may be recorded.

T   **Primary tumor**
TX   Incidental findings of carcinoma in an operative specimen where there had been no previous pre-operative evidence or suspicion of carcinoma
T0   No evidence of primary tumor, but there is evidence of metastases elsewhere
T1   A solitary nodule with a smooth surface occupying less than one lobe of the prostate and surrounded by compressible tissue
T2   A tumor with a smooth surface confined to the prostate and occupying one lobe or more of the prostate
T3   A tumor extending beyond the prostate with or without involvement of the seminal vesicles or the bladder
T4   Tumor fixed to pelvic wall or involving adjoining organs

N   **Regional lymph nodes**
The suffix − (minus) or + (plus) may be added to all N categories according to histological information which may subsequently become available.
NX   When it is not possible to assess the regional lymph nodes
N0   No deformity of regional nodes as shown by available diagnostic measures
N1   Regional nodes deformed as shown by available diagnostic measures
N2   Fixed palpable abdominal nodes

M   **Distant metastases**
For assessment of the M categories the minimum requirements are: (1) chest X-ray, (2) skeletal study (scan or radiography), (3) biochemical tests.

M0 No evidence of distant metastases
M1 Distant metastases present
  M1a Lymph node metastases beyond the regional nodes
  M1b Skeletal metastases
  M1c Visceral metastases
  M1d Pulmonary metastases
  M1e Biochemical evidence of distant metastases, viz. elevated levels of prostatic portion of the serum acid phosphatase on two or more occasions

P Histopathological categories

Three methods are available depending upon the method of obtaining the pathological material, viz. by TUR, by open enucleation or by radical prostatovesiculectomy.

TUR
pX Stage unassessable
p1 Small focus in an otherwise normal gland
p2 Diffuse involvement of all tissue resected

Open enucleation
PX Stage unassessable
P1 Small tumor within adenoma not reaching the edge of enucleation
P2 Diffuse involvement reaching edge of enucleation
P3 Involvement of capsule or vesicles if these have been excised after the enucleation

Radical operation
RPX Stage unassessable
RP1 Involving less than one lobe: no evidence of penetration of capsule
RP2 Involving more than one lobe: no evidence of penetration of capsule
RP3 Involvement of periprostatic tissue, seminal vesicle or bladder neck

G Histopathological grading
GX No information available
G0 Ungradeable
G1 Low grade
G2 Medium grade
G3 High grade

REFERENCES

1. Hudson, P. B. (1957). Prostatic cance XIV. Its incidence, extent and behavior in 686 men studied by prostatic biopsy. *J. Amer. Geriatrics Soc.*, 5, 338
2. Bumpus, H. C. (1926). Carcinoma of the prostate; a clinical study of 1000 cases. *Surgery, Gynecology and Obstetrics*, 43, 150
3. Nesbit, R. M. and Baum, W. C. (1950). Endocrine control of prostatic carcinoma: Clinical and statistical survey of 1818 cases. *J. Amer. Med. Ass.*, 143, 1317

4. Huggins, C. and Hodges, C. V. (1941). Studies on prostatic cancer: I. The effect of castration, of estrogen and of androgen injection on serum phosphatases in metastatic carcinoma of the prostate. *Cancer Res.*, *1*, 292

5. Huggins, C. (1944). The treatment of cancer of the prostate. *Canadian Med. Ass. J.*, *50*, 301

6. Grayhack, J. T. and Wendel, E. F. (1973). Hormone dependence of carcinoma of the prostate. In *Structure and function of male sex accessory organs* (David Brandes, editor). New York: Academic Press

7. Emmett, J. L., Greene, L. F. and Papantoniou, A. (1960). Endocrine therapy in carcinoma of the prostate gland: 10 year survival studies. *J. Urol.*, *83*, 471

8. Franks, L. M. (1967). Carcinoma of Prostate. *Trans. Med. Soc. Lond.*, *83*, 101

9. Franks, L. M., Fergusson, J. D. and Murnaghan, G. F. (1958). An assessment of factors influencing survival in prostatic cancer: the absence of reliable prognostic features. *Brit. J. Cancer*, *12*, 321

10. Schirmer, H. K. A., Murphy, G. P. and Scott, W. W. (1965). Hormonal Therapy prostatic cancer. *Urology Digest*, *4*, 15

11. Schoonees, R., Palma, L. D., Gaeta, J. F., Moore, R. H. and Murphy, G. P. (1972). Prostatic carcinoma treated at categorical center. *N.Y. State J. Med.*, *72*, 1021

12. Prout, G. R. and Brewer, W. R. (1967). Response of men with advanced prostatic carcinoma to exogenous administration of testosterone. *Cancer*, *20*, 1871

13. Smith, P. G., Rush, T. W. and Evans, A. T. (1951). Preliminary report on the clinical use of the Tace (chlorotrianisene) in treatment of prostatic carcinoma. *J. Urol.*, *65*, 886

14. Jonsson, G., Diczfalusy, E., Plantin, L. O., Rohl, L. and Birke, G. (1963). Estradurin (polyestradial phosphate) in treatment of prostatic carcinoma: A clinical and steroid metabolic study. *Acta Endocrinologica*, *44*, (Suppl. 83), 1

15. Geller, J., Fruchtman, B., Newman, H., Robert, T. and Silva, R. (1967). Effect of progestational agents on carcinoma of the prostate. *Cancer Chemotherapy Reports*, *51*, 41

16. Segal, S. J., Marberger, H. and Flocks, R. H. (1959). Tissue distribution of stilbestrol diphosphate: Concentration in prostatic tissue. *J. Urol.*, *81*, 474

17. Fergusson, J. D. (1961). Tracer experiment showing the distribution and fate of injected phosphorylated estrogens in cancer of the prostate. *Brit. J. Urol.*, *33*, 442

18. Lambley, D. G. and Ware, J. W. (1967). Oral stilbestrol diphosphate ("Hovan") in the treatment of prostatic cancer: a clinical trial. *Brit. J. Urol.*, *39*, 147

19. Bergmann, M. (1971). Treatment of prostatic carcinoma. *Acta Chirurgica Austria*, *3*, 100

20. Nilsson, T. and Muntzing, J. (1973). Histochemical and biochemical investigations of advanced prostatic carcinoma treated with estramustine phosphate, estracyt, *Scandinavian J. Urol. Nephrol.*, *7*, 18

21. Jonsson, G. and Hogberg, B. (1971). Treatment of advanced prostatic carcinoma with estracyt. *Scandinavian J. Urol. Nephrol.*, *5*, 103

22. Jonsson, G. (1971). Cytoxic agents in the treatment of prostatic carcinoma. In Life Sciences Monographs 1. *International symposium on the treatment of carcinoma of the prostate*, Berlin Nov. 13–15, 1969. (G. Raspe and W. Brosig, editors). Vieweg: Pergamon Press

23. Herbst, W. P. (1941). The effects of estradiol dipropionate and diethylstilbestrol on malignant prostatic tissue. *Trans. Amer. Ass. Genito-Urinary Surgeons*, *34*, 195

24. Birke, G., Franksson, C. and Plantin, L. O. (1954). On the excretion of androgens in carcinoma of the prostate II. Estrogen therapy before and after orchiectomy. *Acta endocrinologica* (*suppl*), *17*, 1

25. Fergusson, J. D. (1963). Some aspects of the conservative management of prostatic cancer. *Proc. Roy. Soc. Med.*, *56*, 81

26. Fergusson, J. D. (1967). Carcinoma of Prostate. *Trans. Med. Soc. Lond.*, *83*, 92

27. Robinson, M. R. G. and Thomas, B. S. (1971). Effect of hormonal therapy on plasma testosterone levels in prostatic carcinoma. *Brit. Med. J.*, *4*, 391

28. Shearer, R. J., Hendry, W. F. and Fergusson, J. D. (1973). Estrogen treatment in carcinoma of the prostate. *Brit. Med. J.*, *3*, 51 (Letter)

29. Bracci, U. and Di Silverio, F. (1973). Therapeutic procedures in prostatic cancer. Proceedings of 16th Congress International Society of Urology. Amsterdam 1–6 July 1973. To be published by I.S.U.

30. Farnsworth, W. E. (1969). A direct effect of estrogens on prostatic metabolism of testosterone. *J. Invest. Urol.*, *6*, 423

31. Jungblut, P. W., Hughes, S. F., Gorlich, L., Gowers, U. and Wagner, R. K. (1971). Simultaneous occurrence of individual and androgen receptors in female and male target organs. *Hoppe-Seylers Zeitschrift für physiologische Chemie*, *352*, 1603

32. Widmann, B. P. (1934). Cancer of the prostate: The results of radium and roentgen ray treatment. *Radiology*, *22*, 153

33. Flocks, R. H., Culp, D. A. and Elkins, J. B. (1959). Present status of radioactive gold therapy in the management of prostatic cancer. *J. Urol.*, *81*, 178

34. Flocks, R. H. (1963). Combination therapy for localized prostatic cancer. *J. Urol.*, *89*, 889

35. Bulkley, G. J. and O'Connor, V. J. (1960). Carcinoma of the prostate. Treatment by interstitial irradiation with radioactive gold — experimental and clinical studies. *J. Amer. Med. Ass.*, *174*, 252

36. Whitmore, W. F. Jr., Hilaris, B. and Grabstald, H. (1972). Retropubic implantation of Iodine 125 in the treatment of prostatic cancer. *J. Urol.*, *108*, 918

37. Del Regato, J. A. (1967). Radiotherapy in conservative treatment of operable and locally inoperable carcinoma of the prostate. *Radiology*, *88*, 761

38. Bagshaw, M. A., Kaplan, H. S. and Sagerman, R. H. (1965). Linear accelerator supervoltage radiotherapy. VII. Carcinoma of the prostate. *Radiology*, *85*, 121

39. Grout, D. C., Grayhack, J. T., Moss, W. and Holland, J. M. (1971). Radiation therapy in the treatment of carcinoma of the prostate. *J. Urol.*, *105*, 411

40. Bagshaw, M. A. (1973). Primary radiation therapy in cancer of the prostate. Proceedings of 1st National Conference on Urologic Cancer: Washington DC. 29–31 March 1973. To be published by American Cancer Society

41. Carlton, C. E. Jr., Dawould, F., Hudgins, P. and Scott, R. Jr. (1972). Irradiation treatment of the prostate: a preliminary report based on 8 years of experience. *J. Urol.*, *108*, 924

42. Del Regato, J. A. (1973). Radiotherapy as a curative therapy of operable and inoperable carcinoma of the prostate. Proceedings of 16th Congress International Society of Urology, Amsterdam 1–6 July 1973. To be published by I.S.U.

43. Shida, K. (1973). Treatment of prostatic carcinoma by radiologic methods.

Proceedings of 16th Congress of International Society of Urology: Amsterdam 1–6 July 1973. To be published by I.S.U.

44. Smart, J. G. (1965). The use of ^{32}P in the treatment of severe pain from bone metastases of carcinoma of the prostate. *Brit. J. Urol.*, *37*, 139

45. Tong, E. C. K. (1971). Parathormone and radiophosphorus therapy in prostatic cancer with bone metastases. *Radiology*, *98*, 343

46. Hodges, C. V., Moore, R. J., Behnam, A. M. and Lehman, T. H. (1964). Regional perfusion of inoperable prostatic cancer with radioactive phosphorus. *J. Urol.*, *92*, 540

47. Shahmanesh, M., Bolton, C. H., Feneley, R. C. L. and Hartog, M. (1973). Metabolic effects of estrogen treatment in patients with carcinoma of the prostate: A comparison of stilbestrol and conjugated equine estrogens. *Brit. Med. J.*, *2*, 512

48. Byar, D. P. (1973). The V.A. Study of Cancer of the Prostate. Proceedings of 1st National Conference on Urologic Cancer: Washington DC. 29–31 March 1973. To be published by American Cancer Society.

49. Byar, D. P. and V.A.C.U.R.G. (1972). Survival of patients with incidentally found microscopic cancer of the prostate: Results of a clinical trial of conservative treatment. *J. Urol.*, *108*, 908

50. Barnes, R. W. and Ninan, C. A. (1972). Carcinoma of the prostate: Biopsy and conservative therapy. *J. Urol.*, *108*, 897

51. Grayhack, J. T. and Kropp, K. A. (1971). Carcinoma of the Prostate. In *Practice of Surgery*, Chapter 16. (L. Karafin and A. R. Kendell, editors.) Maryland: Harper and Row

52. Baker, R. (1953). Studies on cancer prevention in urology. I. Prostate. *Annals of Surgery*, *137*, 29

53. Byar, D. P. (1972). Treatment of prostatic cancer: studies by V.A.C.U.R.G. *Bull. N.Y. Acad. Med.*, *48*, 751

54. Byar, D. P. (1973). Personal communication

55. Rubin, D. (1969). Cancer of the urinogenital tract: Prostatic cancer. *J. Amer. Med. Ass.*, *210*, 322

6

The radical treatment of prostatic cancer

R. H. Flocks

Introduction

Radical ablation of the local lesion in prostatic cancer is indicated in patients who do not have evidence of dissemination of the lesion and whose life expectancy from the point of view of age and general condition (heart, vessels, lungs, etc.) is five

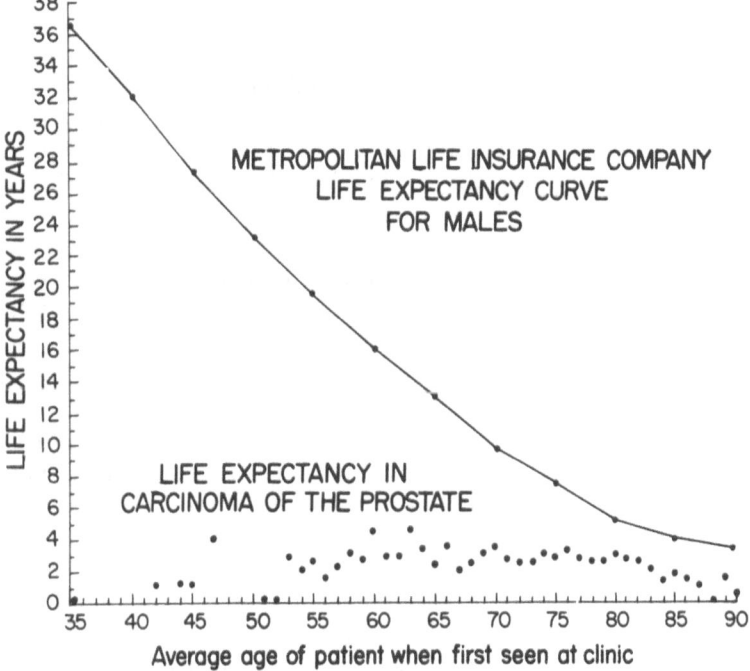

Figure 6.1 Note that conservative therapy for Stage B and C lesions of prostatic cancer is associated with a marked diminution in life expectancy (1294 patients). Each dot represents the average survival for all patients in that age group

y.ears or more. Palliative therapy as seen in Figure 6.1 yields an average of four years and, therefore, is sufficient for those with such a life expectancy; but it is not sufficient for those with a greater life expectancy. It is probable also that in properly selected situations, radical ablation added to palliative therapy will prolong and improve the quality of survival even in the presence of dissemination of the lesion. Careful and meticulous assessment of the patient's general condition and studies such as bone scans, serum acid phosphatase, lymphangiography, cystoscopy and excretory urograms are helpful in making a judgment with regard to the kind of therapy indicated in the individual patient.

The clinical staging of prostatic cancer is discussed in detail in the previous chapter. The Stage 1, or A lesion, is occult. The Stage 2, or B lesion, is completely limited to the prostate and is relatively small. The Stage 3, or C lesion, invades the capsule and the areolar tissue around the prostate itself, around the base of the seminal vesicles and the base of the bladder, with no evidence of lymph node or distant metastasis. This stage includes tumor which was larger than the Stage B lesion, with extensive invasion around the bladder neck and the base of the seminal vesicles, but again with no evidence of metastasis. Stage IV, or 'D' lesions, have vascular metastasis, with or without regional lymph node involvement. This clinical staging is subject to much correction since recent studies indicate that approximately 5% of Stage A and B lesions have either vascular or lymphatic spread, and that of the Stage C lesions, 45% have lymphatic metastases and 5% have vascular metastases. Clinical Stage C comprises approximately 45% of all prostatic cancer seen, with Stages A and B comprising 5% of those seen in practice. It is also clear that only half of these are truly localized to the pelvic area and thus amenable to local destruction.

In addition to the stage, another factor which is extremely important in gaging the prognosis is the microscopic grading. The more aggressive, undifferentiated tumors are more likely to have metastatic lesions and therefore be truly pathologic Stage D lesions. It is also to be emphasized that although the incidence of clinical Stage A and B lesions is only 5% of the patients with prostatic cancer in the usual civilian practice, when careful rectal examinations are carried out in a routine manner (such as can be done in the armed services) the incidence of early prostatic cancer rises tremendously. Kimbrough has shown that this can approximate 50% of all patients with prostatic cancer. Since A and B lesions are readily removed by radical surgery, either by the retropubic or perineal route, it would seem that this would be the standard therapy for these cases. Stage B and C lesions, when treated palliatively, are not associated with a good life expectancy. This is seen in Figure 6.1.

What are the options for the A and B lesions? Since the A and B lesions are limited to the prostate itself, the plane of cleavage around the capsule completely surrounds the lesion and except for the 5% incidence of undiagnosed metastasis to the regional lymph nodes or to the bones, radical removal of the prostate by either the perineal or retropubic route will bring about the complete ablation of the lesion. The results in such cases, as illustrated by Jewett[1], Belt and Schroder[2], and

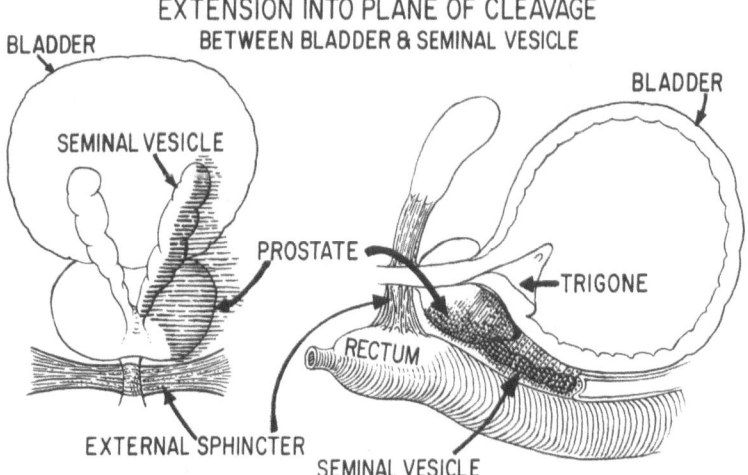

Figure 6.2   Stage C prostatic cancer. Diagram showing extension into plane of cleavage and illustrating the problem of ablation of the local lesion

Culp[3] indicate that the treatment of choice for these lesions is clearly radical prostatectomy. Although the survival rate of Barnes in 15-year group[4] approaches that of Jewett[1] and others, the quality of life is tremendously different. Moreover, a careful study of the statistics indicates that many of Barnes[4] group have been actually cured by the surgical removal of the lesion transurethrally at the time of biopsy, rather than destroyed by general medical hormonal manipulation. There is a definite difference between the quality of survival in Barnes[4] and Jewett's[1] 15-year group, and also a definite possibility that a substantial percentage of the patients described by Barnes[4] were actually surgically ablated by the operative procedure at the time the diagnosis was made.

Radical therapy is still under study for the treatment of Stage C prostatic cancer[5,6]. Here the plane of cleavage for the removal of the local lesion has been invaded either microscopically or grossly by the prostatic cancer, and special maneuvers are necessary to destroy the lesion in the plane of cleavage (Figure 6.2). Also of course the survival rate will be lower, since once the capsule has been penetrated, the incidence of metastatic lesions, particularly to the regional lymph nodes and also to the bones, is significantly increased and may not be discovered prior to the time of institution of local therapy. However, radical prostatectomy plus interstitial irradiation or external irradiation can produce striking results in these 'C' lesions, as indicated by the results of the author. Extended radical surgery can also be utilized for Stage C lesions without the adjuvant therapy of radiation, as illustrated in Figures 6.2–6.6. In the author's opinion[5], the choice between perineal and retropubic prostatectomy is one which should be made in relation to the stage of the lesion and the location of the lesion. If the lesion is Stage C it is best treated through the perineal route for optimal local ablation. In order to make sure that it is a Stage C lesion and not actually a Stage D lesion, it may be necessary to perform pelvic lymphadenectomy. This can be done at the time of the perineal operative procedure, prior to it, or later. A bone scan should be done prior to the operative procedure to rule out osseous metastases. Lymphangiography may also be helpful here, as indicated previously. Elevated serum acid phosphatase should make one suspect the possibility of metastatic lesions.

EXTENDED PROSTATIC REMOVAL
PERINEAL EXPOSURE

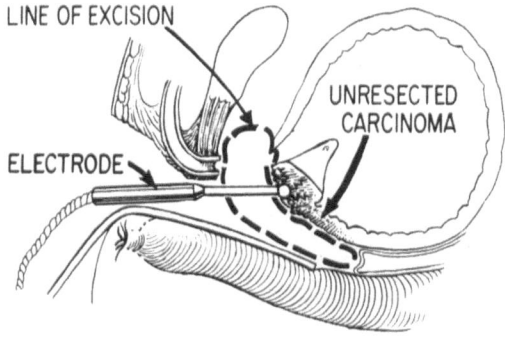

Figure 6.3   Diagram illustrating extended prostatic removal by the perineal route. Note use of electrosurgical coagulation in place of cleavage to destroy spread of cancer in this area

RADICAL PROSTATECTOMY
$+^{198}$Au

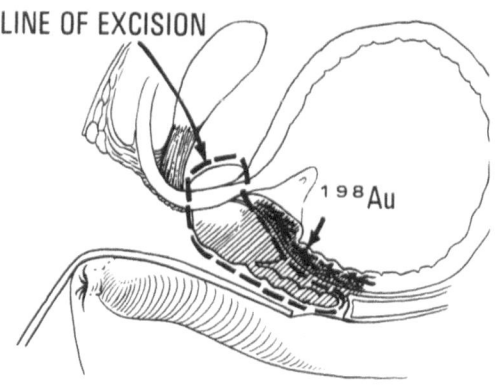

Figure 6.4   Diagram illustrating the use of ^{198}Au injections to destroy residual cancer in the plane of cleavage

EXTENDED PROSTATIC REMOVAL
PERINEAL EXPOSURE

(A)
BLADDER FLAP INCISION

(B)
FLAP ESTABLISHED

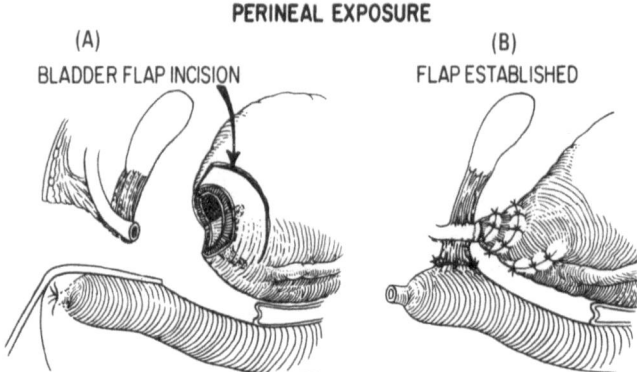

Figure 6.5 Note utilization of spital flap procedure to bridge gap between membranous urethra and bladder neck and preserve continence after extended radical perineal or retropubic prostatectomy

EXTENDED PROSTATIC REMOVAL
RETROPUBIC EXPOSURE

BLADDER
INCISION

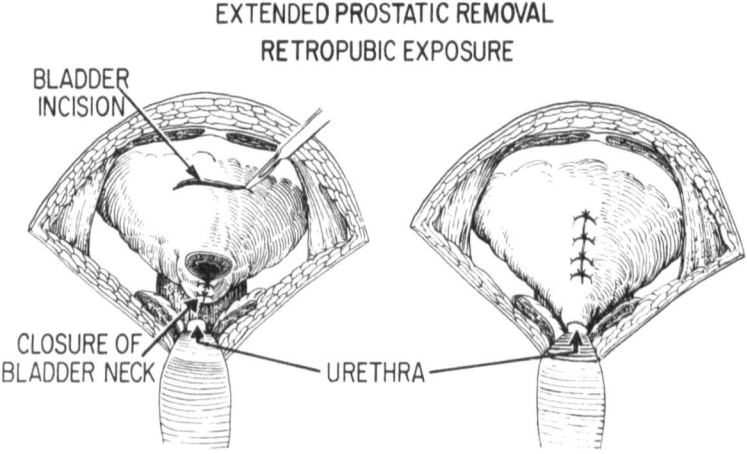

CLOSURE OF
BLADDER NECK   URETHRA

Figure 6.6 Note the use of a transverse incision on the anterior surface of the bladder. It is then sutured longitudinally to enhance the action of the internal sphincter and push the bladder neck cauded to help bridge the gap to the membranous urethra after radical prostatectomy of the extended type

Stage A and B lesions can be treated equally well by either route unless the cancerous lesion is near the apex. If it is, it cannot be as readily excised retropubically as through the perineal route. The advantage of the retropubic route, however, would be to answer definitively the question of regional lymph node involvement.

It is also to be emphasized that surgical excision of the local lesion and adjuvant electrosurgical therapy or irradiation therapy does not exclude the addition of hormonal therapy or bilateral orchiectomy. This combination therapy may add significantly to the management of the individual patient[5] (Tables 6.1–6.5).

Table 6.1 LOCAL RECURRENCE FOLLOWING SURGICAL REMOVAL OF PROSTATIC CANCER WITH EXTRAPROSTATIC EXTENSION. FIVE-YEAR FOLLOW UP

	Number of patients	Number of patients with local recurrence	Percentage
Belt	34	8	21.7
Scott	29	7	21.7
Whitmore and MacKenzie	28	8	28.5
Flocks*	335	15	4.4

* [198]Au used as adjuvant

Comparison of results of radical prostatectomy for C lesions when extended prostatectomy plus adjuvant interstitial radiation is utilized in contrast to ordinary radical surgery. Only a 4.4% incidence of local recurrence was noted after 5 years in contrast to over 20% when no adjuvant therapy was used

Table 6.2 STAGE C CARCINOMA OF THE PROSTATE CLINICAL PATIENTS WITH POSSIBLE LYMPH NODE INVOLVEMENT

No lymphadenectomy, radical prostatectomy, or [198]Au interstitial	
Number of patients	244
Local recurrence	11 (4.5%)
5-Year survival without evidence of tumor	147 (60.7%)

Radical surgery plus interstitial radiation for Stage C cancer

Incidence of local recurrence and survival after 5 years. Status of lymph node involvement unknown

Table 6.3 STAGE C CARCINOMA OF THE PROSTATE—CLINICAL PATIENTS WITHOUT NODE INVOLVEMENT

Radical prostatectomy, lymphadenectomy and [198]Au interstitial	
Number of patients	69
Local recurrence	3 (4.3%)
5-Year survival without evidence of tumor	51 (74%)
10-Year survival without evidence of tumor	44 (66.7%)
15-Year survival without evidence of tumor	19 (27.5%)

Radical surgery for Stage C prostatic cancer. Lymph nodes not involved. Note incidence of local recurrence and survival rate at 5, 10 and 15 years

Table 6.4 IN 384 STAGE B PATIENTS, RETROPUBIC EXPLORATION WAS CARRIED OUT. IN 146 CASES INVOLVEMENT OF THE PELVIC NODES WITHOUT EVIDENCE OF INVOLVEMENT OF ABDOMINAL NODES WAS FOUND. THE OCCURRENCE AS RELATED TO THE SIZE OF THE LESION WAS AS FOLLOWS

Size of local lesion	No. of cases	No. with positive nodes	% with positive nodes
Under 35 g	132	26	20
35–80 g	185	81	44
80–150 g	55	28	51
Larger than 150 g	12	11	92
Totals	384	146	38

During the 6-year period, 29 patients were considered clinically operable. Two of these proved to have positive nodes and were therefore transferred from Group I to Group IIB

Radical perineal prostatectomy

The patient is placed in the exaggerated lithotomy position after the usual primary preparation and draping of the operative field and the placement of an O'Conor shield to make it possible to palpate the position of the rectum throughout the operative procedure. An inverted U-shaped incision is made

Table 6.5 STAGE C CARCINOMA OF THE PROSTATE—CLINICAL PATIENTS WITH LYMPH NODE INVOLVEMENT

Prostatic ablation	Interstitial irradiation + or − prostatectomy	+Lymphadenectomy
Number of patients		32
Local recurrence		1
5-Year survival without evidence of tumor		28
10-Year survival without evidence of tumor	4	
15-Year survival without evidence of tumor	4	

Stage C prostatic cancer with pelvic lymph node involvement. Results after pelvic node removal and radical prostatectomy with adjuvant therapy of interstitial irradiation. Note rapid drop-off in survival between the fifth and tenth year

just above the anus through the skin and subcutaneous tissues (Figure 6.7). The ischiorectal fossa is developed on each side and the central tendon is divided. The rectourethralis muscle is divided. The levator ani are divided on each side to make it possible to pull the rectum down readily. The fascia of Denonvilliers is incised and stripped off the posterior surface of the prostate (Figure 6.8). After the posterior surface of the prostate has been exposed, dissection is carried out from the base of the prostate upward along the outer surface of the seminal vesicles, separating only the rectum and the rectal fascia from the inner layer along the outer surfaces of the seminal vesicles. This can be carried out high up to the very tips of the seminal vesicles by a combination of blunt dissection and some sharp dissection. Then a medium-sized Deaver retractor is inserted between the seminal vesicles and the rectum. If indicated, biopsy of a suspicious lesion can be carried out. From time to time it is important to palpate the rectum to make sure that the correct plane of cleavage is being entered and the rectum is being dissected away satisfactorily from the region of the seminal vesicles. At this time the lateral prostatic vascular pedicles can be readily seen and these can be thoroughly coagulated or suture ligatured, or both, so that some of the blood supply to and from the prostate has been interrupted. Following the mobilization of the entire posterior surface of the

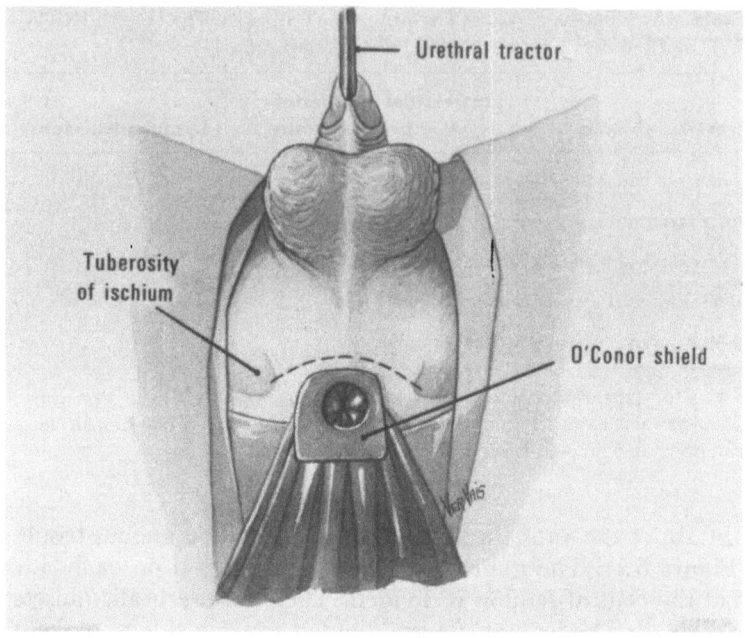

Figure 6.7 This is illustrative of the O'Conor shield in place to make it possible to put a finger in the rectum during the time of perineal exposure. The dotted line shows the inverted V-shaped incision in the perineum. The Lowsley curved tractor is in place

prostate, seminal vesicles and base of the bladder as indicated, the apex of the prostate and lateral surfaces of the prostate are mobilized by a combination of sharp and blunt dissection. The apex of the prostate is divided at its junction with the membranous urethra and a short, straight Lowsley tractor inserted into the prostatic urethra and into the bladder. The blades are opened and then by a combination of sharp and blunt dissection the anterior surface of the prostate and the puboprostatic ligaments are separated from their attachments so that the prostate and bladder neck are thoroughly mobilized and exposed (Figure 6.9). At this point an incision is made on the anterior surface of the bladder neck at its junction with the prostate. This incision is carried around laterally so that the bladder neck can be visualized thoroughly (Figure 6.11). It is important to maintain the bladder neck musculature. There is

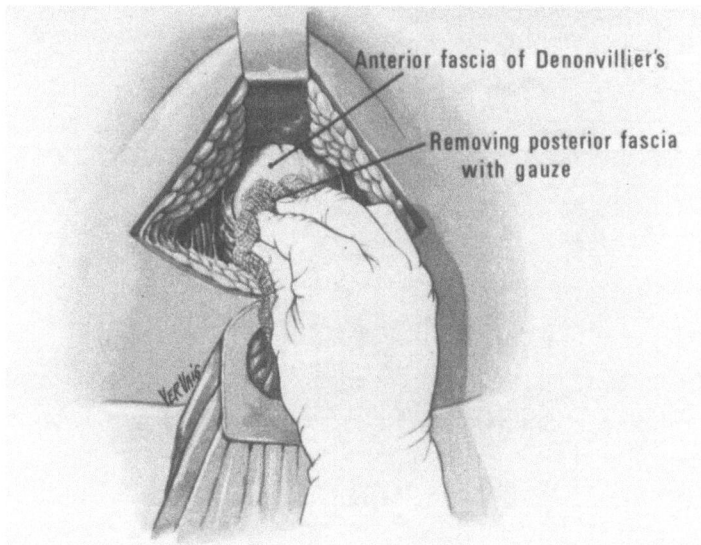

Figure 6.8 The levator ani have been retracted laterally and the rectum posteriorly partially. An incision is made through the posterior layer of Denonvilliers' fascia which then permits easy dissection and separation of the prostate from the rectum down to the base of the seminal vesicle area

a sling of muscle that comes around anteriorly at the bladder neck, which is essentially the internal sphincter (Figure 6.12), and it is important in the maintenance of continence following radical prostatectomy. The urethral orifices can be identified. They can be intubated or their position noted. The incision is then carried on to the posterior bladder neck, through the bladder neck into the subtrigonal tissues. A plane of cleavage is then found between the posterior surface of the bladder and the anterior surface of the seminal vesicles, which is carefully developed along the anterior surface of the seminal vesicles and the vasa deferentia. The vasa deferentia are then divided and suture ligatured. The vascular pedicle is divided and suture ligatured on each side, or coagulated, and the prostate and seminal vesicles along with their surrounding fascia are removed.

The bladder neck is now closed from the posterior surface upward, making sure not to incorporate the ureteral orifices as the closure progresses to the anterior surface of the bladder.

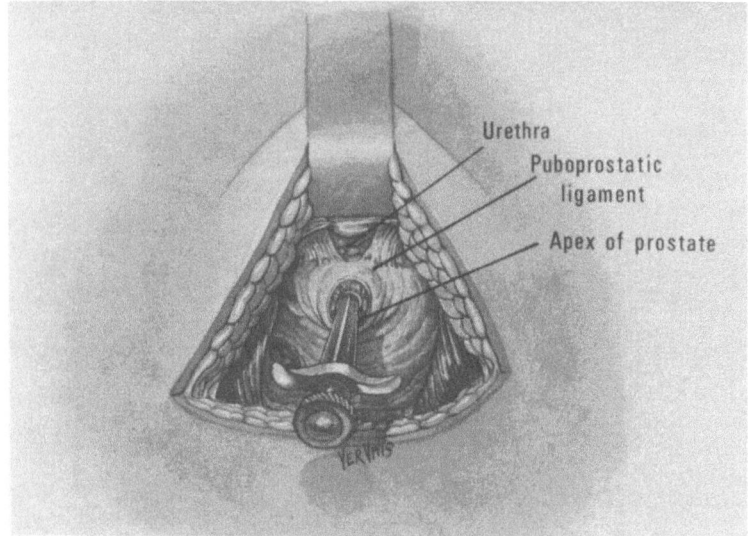

Figure 6.9   Following mobilization of the lateral wall of the prostate and the region of the apex, an incision is made at the apex of the prostate on the long curved Lowsley tractor. Through this the short, straight tractor is inserted and downward traction and outward traction is placed upon the tractor. This brings the apex of the prostate into the wound and visualizes the puboprostatic ligaments which can be divided, thus mobilizing the prostate quite markedly and permitting it to be brought up into the wound

The bladder neck and the sling of muscle in this region—the internal sphincter—is carefully maintained and reconstructed and then approximated with pull-through sutures of size 1 chromic catgut to the membranous urethra so that no sutures are actually placed in the membranous urethra (Figure 6.13). This is done about a 24 French 30 ml Foley catheter. Frequently it has been necessary, in order to completely mobilize the prostate, to incise the levator ani muscles as indicated previously. These are then approximated posteriorly if possible. A small Penrose drain is placed down to the area and the incision closed in two layers with size 00 chromic catgut sutures.

The indwelling urethral catheter is left in place for two weeks. Following its removal the patient is usually partially incontinent, but gradually in the course of the next several

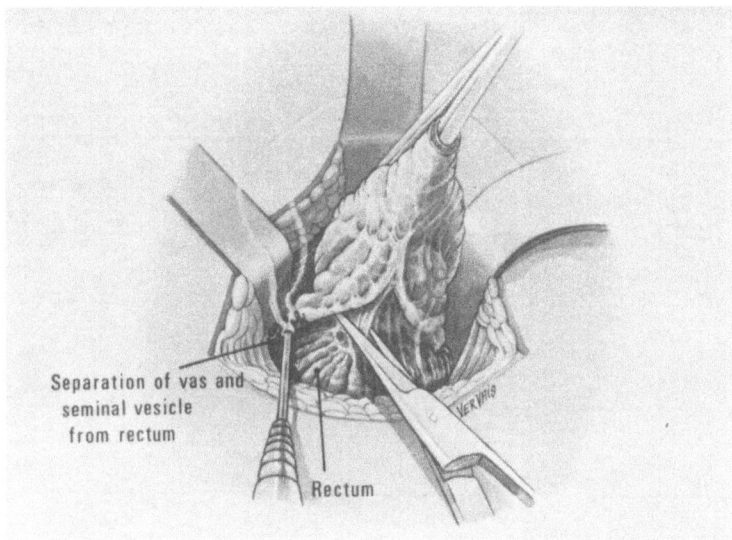

Figure 6.10 The prostate has been mobilized and the posterior surface of the seminal vesicles is being freed right down to their vascular pedicles which are being electrocoagulated

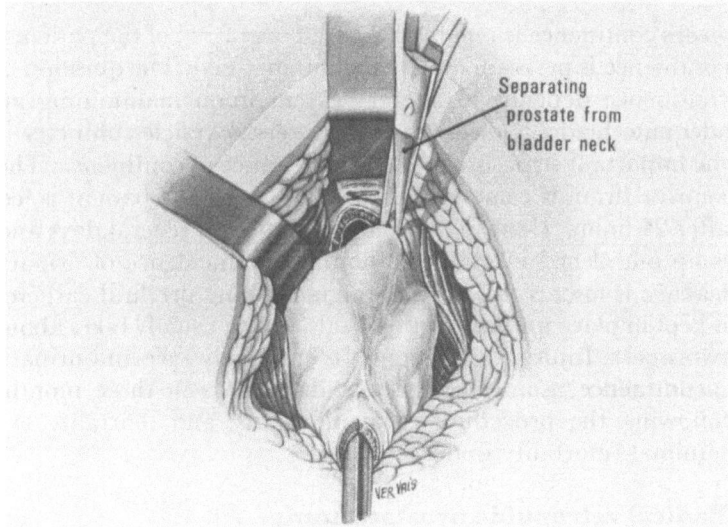

Figure 6.11 The prostate has been markedly mobilized. A small incision is then made on the anterior surface of the neck of the bladder right over the wound as it is visualized

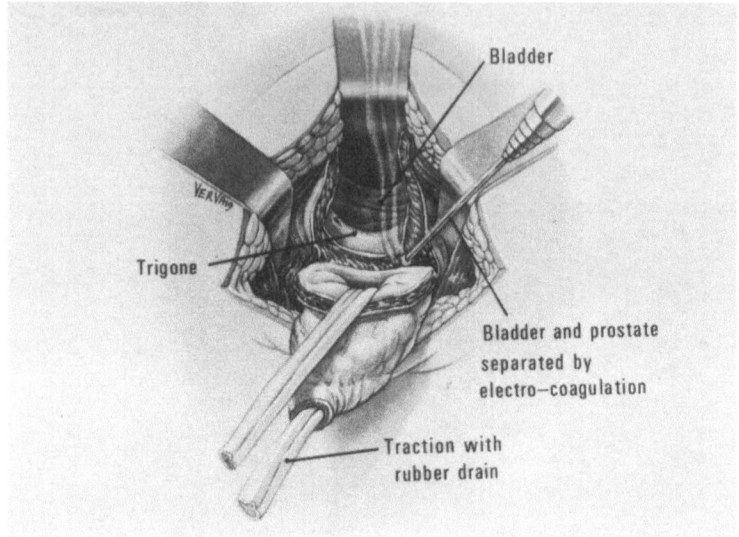

Figure 6.12   This shows further dissection of the anterior neck of the bladder, further separating the prostate from the bladder neck

weeks continence is regained. In well over 95% of the patients, continence is permanent and well maintained. The question of continence depends to a great extent upon maintaining an adequate bladder neck, since the internal vesicle sphincter is the important structure in the maintenance of continence. The Penrose drain is removed on the sixth day. The patient is fed after 24 hours. He is placed on antibiotics for several days and is up out of bed in about 48 hours. The incidence of urinary leakage is low. If this occurs, the indwelling urethral catheter is kept in place until the fistula heals, which usually takes about two weeks. Injury to the rectum is extremely rare and urinary incontinence usually completely disappears in three months following the procedure. The morbidity and mortality are minimal (mortality under 1%).

Radical retropubic prostatectomy
The preoperative care and the anesthesia are the same as for radical perineal prostatectomy. The position on the table, however, is different. The patient is simply placed on his back

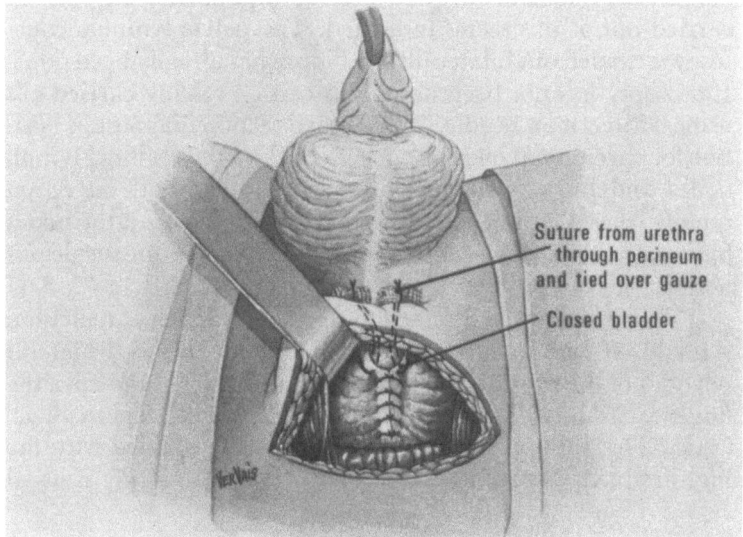

Figure 6.13   The prostatic specimen has been removed. The incision at the bladder neck is well illustrated as is the urethra. The anterior part of the incision is then approximated to the membranous urethra with one or two sutures of size 00 chromic catguts as illustrated. This approximates the area well. The indwelling 24 French, 30 ml Foley Catheter is then inserted into the bladder and the rest of the bladder neck is approximated with size 00 chromic catgut sutures, except for the anterior portions which carry two size 1 chromic catgut sutures which are kept long to be used as tractions sutures and brought through the perineum so that no further sutures are actually utilized, tying the membranous urethra and the bladder neck closely together. The remainder of the bladder neck is approximated with size 00 chromic catgut sutures

with slight elevation of the table underneath the sacrum. The legs are separated slightly so that the penis, scrotum and perineum can be draped into the field. This is important since pull-through sutures are utilized to approximate the bladder neck to the membranous urethra over a urethral catheter.

Having draped the patient satisfactorily, a Czerny incision is made through the skin, subcutaneous tissues, the fascia of the rectus and the recti muscles. The recti muscles are divided close to their insertion into the symphysis pubis, and the incision is carried laterally through the aponeurosis of the external oblique, the internal oblique, and the transversalis muscles so that the entire pelvis can be readily exposed

(Figure 6 14) and an adequate pelvic lymphadenectomy can be carried out, if this seems indicated. The pelvic lymphadenectomy is carried out bilaterally if a biopsy has already been done. If a biopsy has not been done, this can be readily carried out using a Silverman needle. If the frozen section diagnosis is positive for carcinoma, one can then go back to the regional lymph nodes and by a combination of sharp and blunt dissection remove the external iliac, internal iliac and obturator nodes bilaterally. A frozen section can be carried out on suspicious nodes.

Attention is then directed to the prostate itself. An incision is made through the pelvic fascia on either side and the lateral portions of the prostate are freed (Figure 6.15). At the apex the finger is insinuated between the two layers of Denonvilliers' fascia. The puboprostatic ligaments are then divided with the high frequency current (Figure 6.16). Venous oozing is usual

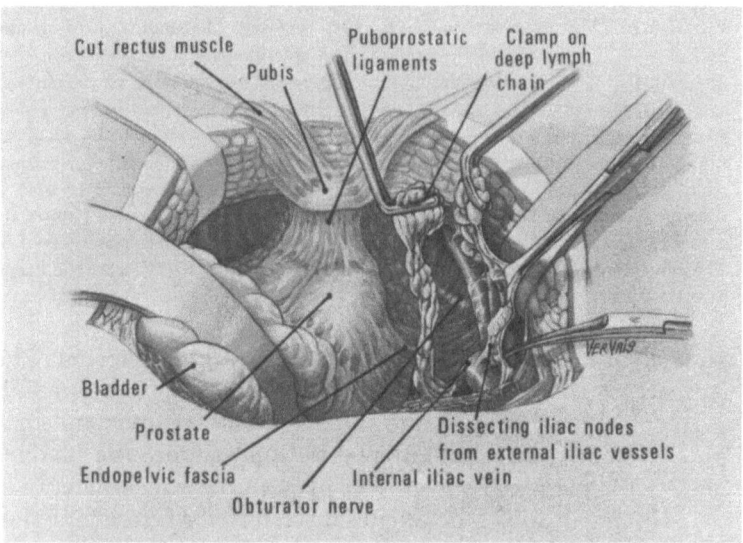

Figure 6.14 The pelvic area has been exposed retropubically. The pelvic node dissection is in progress. Following the node dissection the endopelvic fascia on each side of the prostate will be incised and the prostate partially mobilized. Then puboprostatic ligaments are divided, the urethra is divided and a 30 ml Foley bag placed through the distal urethra, the bag blown up and pulled down. This controls the bleeding in the pelvis

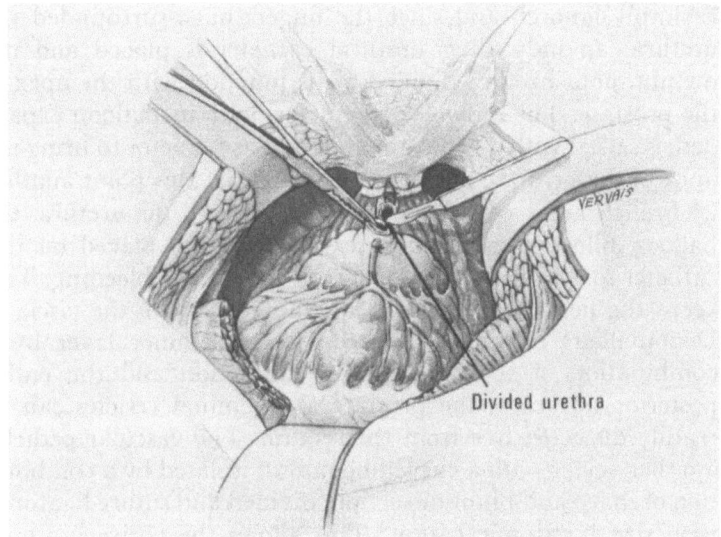

Figure 6.15   The urethra being divided

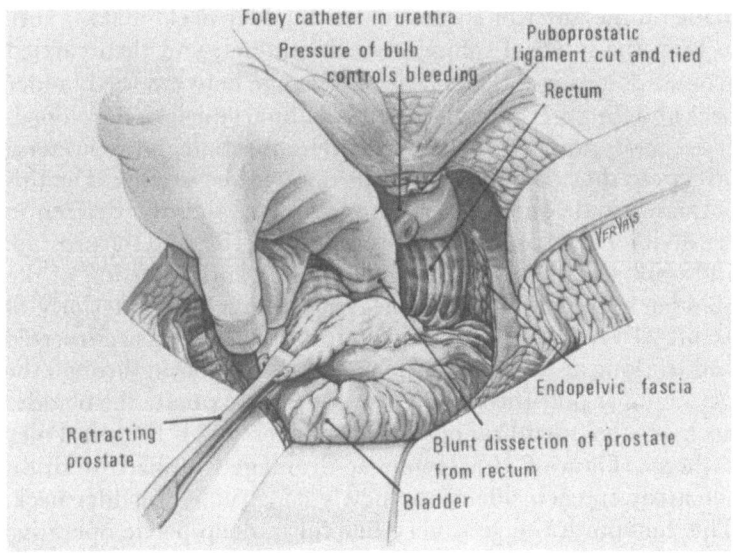

Figure 6.16   The prostate being separated from the rectum. Note how Foley catheter controls bleeding in the pelvis

and cannot be controlled by ligature. At this point, bleeding is simply ignored and since the fingers have surrounded the urethra, an indwelling urethral catheter is placed and the membranous urethra divided at its junction with the apex of the prostate. The indwelling catheter, with its balloon expanded, is seized with a hemostat and used as a tractor to bring the apex of the prostate up into the wound. At this point another 24 French Foley catheter is inserted through the urethra, the balloon filled with 40 ml water and traction placed on this catheter so that the balloon controls the venous bleeding. This keeps the field perfectly dry. The outer layer of the fascia of Denonvilliers is then separated from the inner layer by a combination of sharp and blunt dissection and the entire posterior surface of the prostate and seminal vesicles can be readily dissected free from the rectum. The vascular pedicles are then seized with a curved hemostat, isolated by a combination of sharp and blunt dissection, divided and suture ligatured with size 1 chromic catgut. This allows the entire prostate, seminal vesicles and posterior surface of the bladder to be brought up into the wound (Figure 6.17). An incision is then made on the anterior surface of the bladder neck, making sure to keep the internal sphincteric sling intact, and then carried around posteriorly. The plane of cleavage between the bladder neck and the anterior surface of the seminal vesicles is developed. It is good practice at this point to intubate both ureteral orifices so that no damage will be done to the ureters. The tips of the seminal vesicles are suture ligatured, the vasa deferentia are divided and suture ligatured (Figure 6.18), and the prostate and seminal vesicles thus removed. The entire portion of the bladder neck is then closed, leaving an opening anteriorly of about 24 French. Three 1 chromic catgut sutures are inserted and left long at the bladder neck. These are placed through the perineum as pull-through ligatures to approximate the bladder neck to the membranous urethra over a 24 French Foley catheter (Figure 6.19). Hemovac drainage is utilized to drain the areas on each side of the newly constructed bladder neck. This suction drainage is very helpful in deep pelvic operative procedures. The incision is closed in layers after suturing the recti to their insertion in the symphysis pubis. The rectus fascia and the various muscle layers are approximated with size 1

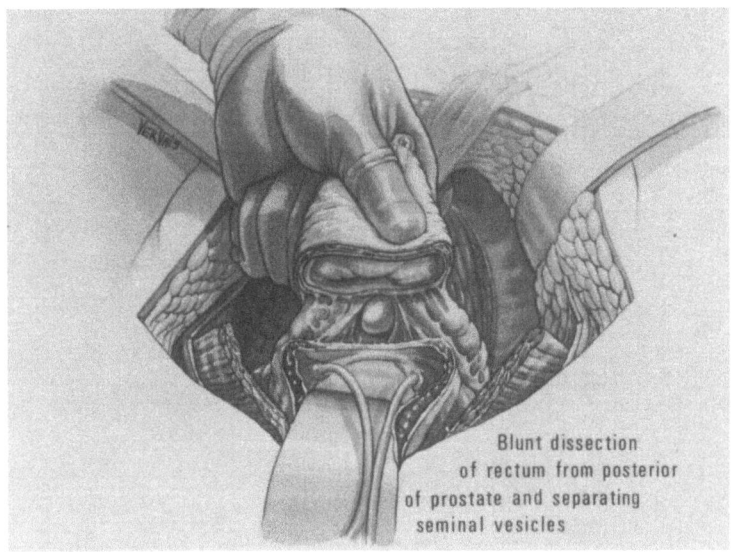

Figure 6.17   Further dissection of prostate and seminal vesicles and their fascia

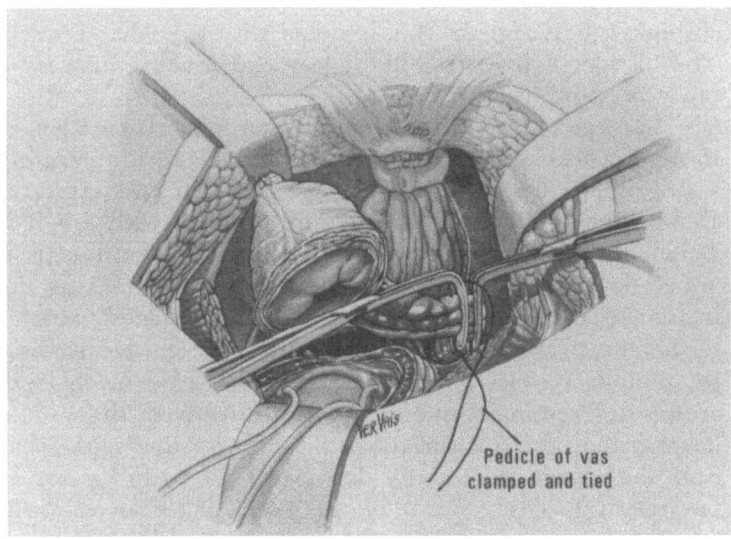

Figure 6.18   The seminal vesicle pedicle being clamped prior to removal of the entire specimen

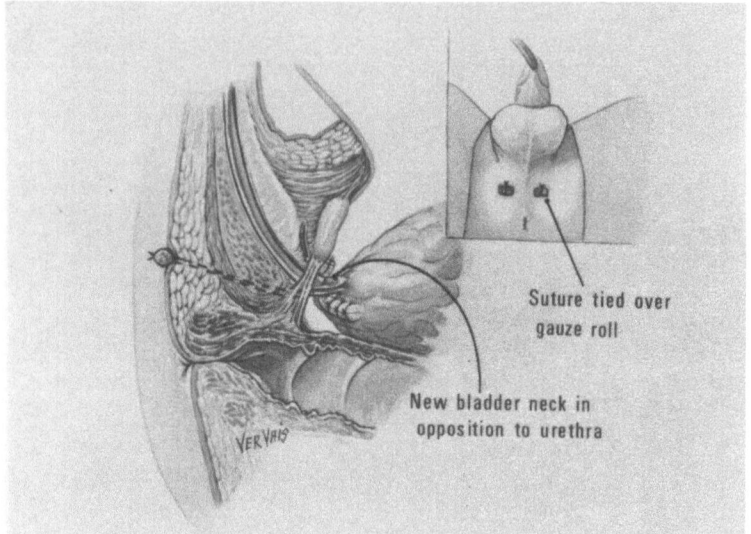

Suture tied over
gauze roll

New bladder neck in
opposition to urethra

VERVHIS

Figure 6.19   The anastomosis of bladder neck to urethra over catheter, utilizing pull-through sutures

chromic catgut and the skin is closed with size 0000 Tevdek. The bladder is irrigated thoroughly and usually there is no problem with bleeding.

Damage to the rectum is extremely rare if care is taken at the time of development of the apex of the prostate in separating and gaining the plane of cleavage between two layers of Denonvilliers' fascia. If there is any problem with this it is usually wise to attack the posterior surface of the prostate from above downward. This can be done by simply making the incision at the bladder neck first, cutting completely around the bladder neck, and developing the plane of cleavage between the seminal vesicles and the bladder. Having done this, get around the seminal vesicles and then directly in the middle develop the posterior surface of the prostate and separate it from the rectum from above downward. This can be carried out relatively easily down to the apex, and then this will facilitate further separation of the two layers of Denonvilliers' fascia at the apex. If the rectum has been entered, meticulous closure, perineal suction drainage, and marked dilatation of the anal sphincter are instituted. A low residue diet is instituted post-operatively for seven to eight days. Pull through of the proximal rectum, as carried out in the Young–Stone procedure, may be valuable in this situation. Injury to the rectum is extremely rare if care is taken in the dissection at the apex of the prostate.

The post-operative care is quite simple. We leave the suction drainage for about six to seven days. The bladder is kept thoroughly irrigated. The patient is placed on intravenous antibiotics. The diet is gradually increased to a regular diet by the sixth or seventh day. The indwelling catheter is kept in place for two weeks. Thereafter there is usually some incontinence which gradually improves and usually by the end of the third month complete continence is present. Again, the matter of continence here depends upon the meticulous closure and maintenance of the internal sphincteric mechanism.

Combination therapy for Stage C prostatic carcinoma

Table 6.6 illustrates the options available for local ablation of a lesion in Stage C carcinoma of the prostate. There is evidence that such ablation, combined with bilateral orchiectomy or estrogen therapy, or both, is definitely superior in the survival of the patient as compared to palliative therapy alone, since in many patients (approximately 50%) no metastases are present and when they are, local problems are eliminated by ablation of the tumor.

The work of Bagshaw[7], particularly, shows the important effects of external irradiation in Stage C carcinoma. Although he reports a 13% local recurrence rate in all types of lesions, and others such as Rhamy et al.[8] report up to 85% local recurrence, his results indicate that serious consideration should be given to external irradiation in selected cases. In the author's experience combined extended radical perineal prostatectomy, plus adjuvant radiation interstitially results in a much lower incidence of local recurrence (see Tables 6.1–6.3). In some of these cases it is important to carry out very carefully and meticulously plastic surgery at the bladder neck to prevent incontinence. The operative procedure developed by the author consists of the development of a spiral-flap closure of the

Table 6.6 TREATMENT OPTIONS FOR STAGE C PROSTATIC CANCER

Palliation: endocrine therapy

Radical prostatectomy and seminal vesiculectomy

Extended radical prostatectomy

Radical pelvic surgery

External radiation

Interstitial radiation

Combination of above

---

bladder neck and is important in preventing incontinence when radical surgery is carried out on the prostate[9].

The presence of involved lymph nodes alters the prognosis significantly. Trials are being carried out at the present time with regard to radiation therapy of the regional lymph nodes. Regional lymph node removal in a series of 32 patients carried out in 1954 and followed for 15 years or more would seem to indicate that when lymph nodes are positive, although local recurrence does not occur frequently, the incidence of vascular metastasis is so high at the time the procedure is carried out that only a 12%, 15-year survival is probable (see Tables 6.4 and 6.5).

The cryosurgical destruction of Stage C prostatic carcinoma through the perineal route has shown strikingly good results in a small number of cases undergoing a preliminary trial of this modality[10]. Figure 6.20 shows the prostatic cancer exposed perineally and the cryoprobe in contact with the carcinomatous tissue and destroying it. The extent of the destruction and the nature of the repair has been very satisfactory. The prostatic urethra has not been destroyed, continence has not been interfered with, and the wound has healed relatively rapidly with a good deal of drainage through a perineal sinus which has cleared up in about five or six weeks. Some general effects have been noted. The reason for this is not yet clear, but the possibility of immunological effects is being intensively studied.

In summary, then, the following may be stated: Evidence has been presented for utilization of radical ablation of a local

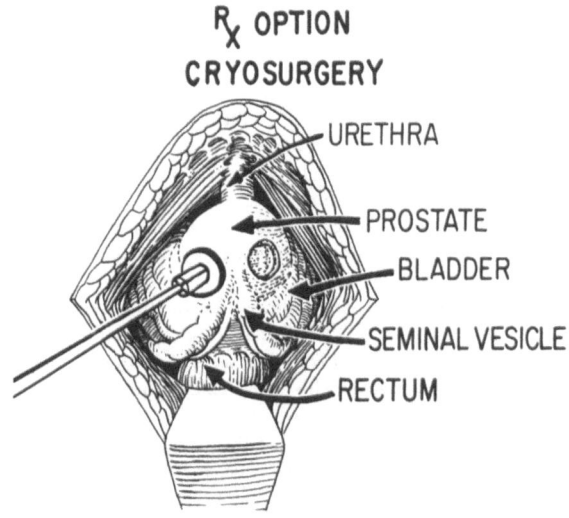

Figure 6.20   Showing the use of the cryosurgical probe to destroy the prostatic cancer through a perineal incision

lesion for prostatic cancer in those who have a general life expectancy of over 5 years and no evidence of dissemination of the lesion. The presence of positive lymph nodes produces a poor prognosis. Although the local lymph nodes are either removed or destroyed by combinations of surgery and irradiation, metastasis to the bones show up in the course of the life history of the lesion so that a 15-year survival rate of not more than 10 or 12% seems possible.

The techniques for local ablation have been listed and briefly described, including external irradiation alone (Bagshaw[7]), interstitial alone or with radical prostatectomy (Flocks[11]), radical prostatectomy, both perineal and retropubic, extended radical prostatectomy (Flocks[5]), combination radical prostatectomy and cryosurgical prostatectomy.

REFERENCES

1. Jewett, H. J. (1970). The case for radical prostatectomy. *J. Urol.*, *103*, 195
2. Belt, E. and Schroder, F. H. (1972). Total perineal prostatectomy for carcinoma of the prostate. *J. Urol.*, *107*, 91

3. Culp, O. S. (1967). Radical perineal prostatectomy: Its past, present and future. *J. Urol.*, *98*, 618

4. Barnes, R. W. (1953). Results of palliative treatment of early carcinoma of the prostate. *J. Urol.*, *70*, 489

5. Flocks, R. H. (1973). The treatment of Stage C prostatic cancer with special reference to combined surgical and radiation therapy. *J. Urol.*, *109*, 461

6. Vickery, A. L. and Kerr, W. S. (1963). Carcinoma of the prostate treated by radical prostatectomy: A clinocopathological survey of 187 cases followed for 5 years and 148 cases followed for 10 years. *Cancer*, *16*, 1598

7. Bagshaw, M. A. (1969). Definitive radiotherapy in carcinoma of the prostate. *J. Amer. Med. Ass.*, *210*, 326

8. Rhamy, R. K., Wilson, S. K. and Caldwell, W. L. (1972). Biopsy-proved tumor following definitive irradiation for resectable carcinoma of the prostate

9. Flocks, R. H. and Boldus, R. (1973). The surgical treatment and prevention of urinary incontinence associated with disturbance of the internal urethral sphincteric mechanism. *J. Urol.*, *109*, 279

10. Flocks, R. H. and Nelson, C. M. K. and Boatman, D. L. (1972). Perineal cryosurgery for prostatic carcinoma. *J. Urol.*, *108*, 933

11. Flocks, R. H. (1963). Combination therapy for localized prostatic cancer. *J. Urol.*, *89*, 894

7

Adrenalectomy and hypophysectomy in disseminated prostatic cancer

W. F. Hendry

Introduction

The misery of the patient with advanced prostatic cancer often presents a formidable problem in urological practice. Extensive local growth leads to increasing difficulty with micturition and metastases in bone may produce the most intolerable pain. Estrogen therapy or orchidectomy can produce dramatic and long lasting improvement in the previously untreated case, but eventual relapse is almost inevitable.

It is a widely held view that there is little that can be offered to the patient once this stage has been reached, apart from analgesics to ease the discomfort in the weeks before his death. In this chapter, we shall consider the results that have been reported with adrenalectomy and hypophysectomy in the terminal stages of this disease and try to assess whether such a major assault on the endocrine system is a practical and worthwhile proposition.

Historical aspects

In 1941, Huggins et al.[1] reported the results of orchidectomy in 21 patients with advanced prostatic cancer: four patients died shortly afterwards, but all except three of the survivors showed a noticeable improvement in their clinical state. In a further report, Huggins and Hodges[2] observed that the acid phosphatase in cases with bone metastases was markedly reduced by this procedure and by stilbestrol 1 mg/day, but rose with testosterone. In considering these results, they suggested that androgens could also be produced in varying amounts or activity in extragonadal sites.

Further evidence for this was provided by Scott and Vermuelen in 1942[3], who showed that although castration led at first to a fall in urinary 17-ketosteroids, the levels subsequently rose and they also observed a rise in urinary gonadotrophins. These observations were confirmed by Dean et al.[4] who showed in addition that stilbestrol 1 mg/day diminished both urinary 17-ketosteroids and gonadotrophins.

In an attempt to remove extragonadal androgens, Huggins and Scott[5] in 1944 performed bilateral adrenalectomy in four patients with advanced prostatic cancer. The first two cases died in shock at 36 and 54 hours; case 3 died at 11 days; but case 4 survived with adrenocortical extract and deoxycorticosterone acetate for 116 days. His pain was relieved and marked reduction of urinary 17-ketosteroids was observed. Urinary androgens (measured by the chick-comb growth assay) were absent. In 1947, Cox[6] performed left adrenalectomy in two cases without effect, but observed transient improvement in a third patient with paraplegia following total left and four-fifths right adrenalectomy.

With the introduction of cortisone into clinical practice in 1950[7], bilateral adrenalectomy could be performed more safely, and in 1951, Huggins and Bergenstal[8] reported a further two cases who underwent bilateral adrenalectomy during relapse after previous orchidectomy and estrogen therapy. Both patients showed marked improvement: their pain was relieved, their weight increased and they returned to work.

The role of the pituitary in the control of prostatic cancer was being investigated at this time, both experimentally and clinically, by W. W. Scott and colleagues[9–12]. They observed that the prostate glands of hypophysectomised, castrated rats were less responsive to the same dose of testosterone than prostates of castrated rats with intact pituitaries[9]. Prolactin, ACTH, thyroxin, cortisone and gonadotrophin were investigated and it was concluded that prolactin was the main factor which augmented the effects of testosterone[13]. The first surgical hypophysectomy for advanced prostatic cancer was performed in 1948, but the patient died after 11 days. Again the introduction of cortisone allowed this operation to receive further trial and in 1954, Scott reported that five further cases had undergone this procedure: these patients survived for 2 days, 1 month and 3 days, 5 months and 10 days, 9 months and 11 days, and 1 year and 23 days. At autopsy some residual pituitary tissue was found in all cases. Two patients with a small residue had had a good clinical response: in one case there was marked local tumor regression and a pathological fracture healed in the second case. Two patients with a considerable pituitary residue had no response. Marked atrophy of adrenals and testes was noted and the tumor itself showed atrophy and persisting cancer side-by-side[11].

Following these early studies, bilateral adrenalectomy was extensively used in the management of advanced prostatic and breast cancer, and increasingly ingenious methods of pituitary ablation were devised and then subjected to clinical trial.

The adrenals
BILATERAL ADRENALECTOMY

In most reported series, this procedure was done late in the course of the disease, once castration and estrogen therapy had failed. Experience with its effects at an earlier stage are therefore limited, although Morales et al.[14] reported rather disappointing results in nine previously untreated patients, of whom only two obtained complete and three partial relief of pain; four were unchanged and there was no objective evidence of regression. More recently Schoonees et al.[15] reported good response in all six patients who received combined castration with bilateral adrenalectomy as primary treatment, but it is difficult to distinguish the effects of adrenalectomy from orchidectomy in these cases. Certainly there seems to be no evidence in favor of undertaking major endocrine ablation at an early stage in the disease.

The operative approach to the adrenals has been considered in detail by a number of authors[16,17]. In 1952, Huggins and Bergenstal reported 29 cases of simultaneous bilateral adrenalectomy with no immediate mortality[18], but most have preferred to stage the procedure, allowing two weeks between the operations on one side and the other. With modern anesthetic techniques, simultaneous operation should be possible in most cases and in a recent report[19] only three of twenty-two cases were considered to be in such poor general condition that the procedure had to be staged. Most authors have favored a loin approach through the bed of the 11th or 12th rib, but Scardino et al.[20] used a bilateral posterior approach modified from Young's technique[21] in order to avoid turning the patient.

Steroid supportive therapy during and after adrenalectomy has varied, but a regime similar to that recommended by Thorn *et al.*[22] has generally been used and found to be reliable[23]. This comprises cortisone 100 mg i.m. 12 and 2 hours pre-operatively, supplemented by hydrocortisone 10 mg/hour intravenously during and for 4–6 hours after operation. Cortisone is then given intravenously in a dose of 50 mg 6 hourly on post-operative day 1, 50 mg 8 hourly on days 2 and 3, 50 mg 12 hourly on days 4 and 5 and then 25 mg 6 hourly by mouth from day 6, reducing to a maintenance dose of 37.5–50 mg daily. An adequate salt intake is essential and 3–6 g of sodium chloride may have to be added to the diet to ensure an intake of at least 80 mEq/day[22,23]. There is good evidence[24] that the dose of cortisone should not exceed the minimum required for maintenance, since the urinary androgen excretion has been shown to rise if more than 100 mg of cortisone is given daily and to approach normal levels if the dose reaches 300 mg daily.

Table 7.1 SUMMARY OF SOME EARLY PUBLISHED RESULTS OF BILATERAL ADRENALECTOMY IN PATIENTS WITH ADVANCED PROSTATIC CANCER

Author and year (Ref.)	Number of cases	Improvement Subjective	Improvement Objective*
Huggins and Bergenstal[18]	4	4	4
West et al.[25]	10	7	2
Baker[26,27]	10	6	0
Butler et al.[28]	2	2	0
Harrison et al.[29]	7	5	1
Scardino et al.[20]	3	2	1
Birke et al.[30]	11	7	—
Morales et al.[14]	18	9(BNO†)	1
Morales et al.[14]	10	4(Pain†)	1
Pyrah[16]	7	1	0
Fergusson[31]	13	11	—
Macfarlane et al.[17]	13	9	—

* Criteria for objective evidence of remission varied from series to series—see text
† In this series, 9 of 18 patients with symptoms of bladder neck obstruction and 4 of 10 patients with bone pain showed subjective improvement

Some early clinical results obtained with bilateral adrenalectomy are summarised in Table 7.1. In general, about half the patients showed significant subjective improvement, but objective evidence of tumor regression was much less common. Although local prostatic shrinkage on rectal examination, diminished acid phosphatase levels and weight gain were often observed[18], radiological signs of tumor regression were exceptional. Pyrah[16] commented, "It is not known why the results of adrenalectomy for metastatic prostatic cancers are inferior to those of metastatic mammary cancers when the rationale of the operation appears to be the same. The radiographs of the metastates do not always show the striking response seen in successfully treated cases of cancer of the breast, even when there appears to have been a clinical response". However, Franks[32] did observe massive central necrosis of primary and secondary tumors in a patient dying six weeks after bilateral adrenalectomy.

Harrison et al.[29,30] demonstrated that urinary androgens (measured by the chick-comb assay), which had been sharply diminished by castration, were still further reduced to a minimal level by adrenalectomy. However, they did note that complete elimination was not accomplished. Birke et al.[30] measured urinary androgen excretion (androsterone and etiocholanolone) and observed that although orchidectomy reduced the levels by 60%, they subsequently rose again within one month to reach or exceed pre-operative levels in more than 50% of patients. Total suppression could be achieved by stilbestrol 30 mg/day, cortisone 50–75 mg daily, or by castration and bilateral adrenalectomy. They found that a good clinical response correlated well with reduction in these hormones. Burt et al.[34] confirmed these observations and suggested that adrenalectomy should be reserved for those patients with demonstrably high urinary androgen metabolites whilst receiving cortisone therapy.

The mortality rate was high in some of these early published series. West et al.[25] described three post-operative deaths in ten patients, Morales et al.[14] two deaths in twenty cases and Fergusson[31] reported that six of nineteen cases died before the therapeutic response could be evaluated.

The enthusiasm that was expressed in some early reports

gradually declined especially after Pearson et al.[35] demonstrated significant quantities of accessory adrenal tissue in 32% of 100 autopsies and, after describing clinical experience with 12 patients, concluded: "Adrenalectomy for advanced prostatic cancer as presently carried out is not a practical therapeutic procedure". In 1956, Whitmore[36] expressed disappointment in the results of adrenalectomy: the subjective improvement observed in about half of the patients was short lived and unpredictable and objective remission occurred in less than 10%. Similarly Ray[37] in 1957 wrote: "The benefits of adrenalectomy are so meagre and of such short duration as to discourage any further use of it. We have been so discouraged ... that we have not used adrenalectomy for more than two years". Nevertheless, he concluded: "Yet I wonder if there may not be an occasional patient for whom this procedure would be worthwhile."

The problem of identification of the patient who might benefit from adrenalectomy has stimulated further interest in adrenalectomy in recent years. Mahoney and Harrison[19] studied the results obtained with 22 patients in relapse following treatment with estrogens, castration and cortisone inhibition. There were no operative deaths, although in 19 cases the procedure was performed in one stage. Survival ranged from 4–46 months (mean 13 months), which compared favorably with the average of 9–10 months for patients with reactivated disease. Patients were subdivided into two groups on the basis of length of survival (Group 1 less than 10 months —mean 7 months; Group 2 more than 10 months—mean 22 months). Retrospective analysis showed no significant difference in age or length of history in the two groups. Patients that showed the best response appeared to be those who were least anemic, had higher acid phosphatases and had had the longest interval between castration and adrenalectomy. The longest survival (20, 25 and 46 months) was recorded in patients whose tumors were well differentiated. There was no distinct correlation between the results of adrenalectomy and the previous response to cortisone suppression (vide infra). Two patients who had no response to cortisone, even though urinary 17-ketosteroids fell, had a good response after adrenalectomy; and three cases which improved with medical treatment were not improved by surgery. Overall, 81% of patients experienced some subjective benefit and objective evidence of remission was observed in 36%. This article concludes by describing a bed-ridden patient who was so improved after adrenalectomy that he was able to track a bear for several miles, shoot and skin the beast and then aid in transporting the 300 pound carcass to his home five miles away.

Additional experience with adrenalectomy was also reported in 1972 from the Roswell Park Memorial Institute. Schoonees et al.[15] compared the response to adrenalectomy in three groups of patients. Group 1 comprised six patients in relapse after previous estrogen-castration and hypophysectomy —only one showed a transient subjective response; in Group 2, three of thirteen patients in relapse after previous estrogen-castration showed complete response; and in Group 3 six previously untreated patients all responded to orchidectomy followed by adrenalectomy within three months. The endocrine response to adrenalectomy was defined in this paper and in a further communication by Reynoso and Murphy[38]. Eight previously orchidectomised patients were studied before and one and three months after adrenalectomy. Plasma testosterone remained unchanged between 40 and 50 ng/100 ml. Total urinary ketosteroids were moderately diminished; fractionation showed that the 11-deoxy-17-ketosteroids (androgenic fraction) were significantly lowered while the 11-oxy-17-ketosteroids (non-androgenic fraction) were approximately doubled. Gonadotrophin assay showed that both LH and FSH were raised post-operatively (LH significantly raised), suggesting that there may be a negative adrenal/pituitary gonadotrophin feedback.

These additional reports confirmed that some patients derived considerable benefit from bilateral adrenalectomy, but a clear cut method of case selection is still lacking. The endocrine studies showed that this procedure would significantly alter the hormone environment of the tumor but consistently suggested that it should be possible to achieve a similar effect by suppressive drug therapy.

ADRENAL SUPPRESSION

Bilateral adrenalectomy is a major operation to inflict upon a patient already ill with disseminated cancer. The possibility that a similar response could be obtained by medical suppression of adrenal function by cortisone therapy was therefore investigated. In 1954, Valk and Owens[39] reported results obtained with twelve patients with bone metastases, in relapse after previous orchidectomy and estrogen therapy. Cortisone was given in high dosage: 300 mg/day for up to 61 days and then 100 mg daily for up to 76 days, followed by a maintenance dose of 25–50 mg daily together with stilbestrol 5 mg daily. All patients experienced subjective relief of pain, with increased vigor and activity, X-ray evidence of regression of secondary tumor in bone was seen in one case and the acid phosphatase dropped in all eight cases in whom it had previously been elevated. Survival ranged from 3 to 75 months (average 20.2 months). Side effects were serious with such high doses of cortisone—seven patients died, from pneumonia, thrombosis, tuberculosis, congestive cardiac failure, or from stopping the cortisone abruptly. Two of the survivors developed heart failure and one bled from peptic ulcer. Urinary 17-ketosteroids were noted to be high when the patients were receiving the large doses, but low on maintenance doses of cortisone.

Munson et al.[24] studied the effects of the dose of cortisone on urinary 17-ketosteroid excretion and androgen activity in adrenalectomised, orchidectomised patients with prostatic cancer and showed no significant increase in androgen excretion with cortisone doses of 25–50 mg daily; the level increased if the dosage exceeded 100 mg daily, and reached near normal levels with 300 mg daily.

Miller and Hinman[40] treated ten patients with 50–100 mg daily doses of cortisone: eight showed marked subjective improvement, of whom one returned to full work on a cattle ranch; objective improvement with decrease in the size of the local lesion was noted in six; and acid phosphatase declined in two cases. The average duration of response was 82 days (maximum six months). There appeared to be little relationship between clinical improvement and change in urinary 17-ketosteroids.

Birke et al.[30] observed an excellent response in three, very good in three, good in two and no response in four, of twelve patients treated with 50–75 mg of cortisone daily. They found that this dose of cortisone depressed urinary androgen activity completely in most cases and considered that the clinical effect correlated well with reduction in hormones.

Aminoglutethimide was introduced as a treatment for petit mal epilepsy, but its use was discontinued as it appeared to produce adrenal suppression. Recently Robinson *et al.*[41] have used this drug in the treatment of 26 patients with advanced prostatic cancer, supplemented by cortisone 25–50 mg daily, as replacement therapy. About 60% of cases showed subjective improvement, but very few showed objective evidence of tumor regression. The duration and extent of response appeared to be less than with pituitary ablation and side effects, including depression, were sometimes troublesome.

Despite the simplicity of medical suppression of adrenal function and the definite though often short-lived subjective improvement that has been described, this treatment is seldom used in clinical practice at present. The evidence summarised above suggests that further trials of this form of therapy are warranted.

The pituitary

Dissatisfaction with the clinical results achieved with bilateral adrenalectomy led several investigators to transfer their attention away from the adrenals toward the pituitary. There seemed to be a number of good reasons for doing so. Effective destruction of the pituitary should produce complete adrenal suppression, regardless of the possible existence of functionally important accessory adrenal tissue, which had been found in 32% of 100 autopsies[35]. Gonadotrophins would be destroyed at source. Furthermore, considerable experimental evidence had suggested that prolactin might be concerned with prostatic growth[9]. Further studies showed that radioactive labeled prolactin was concentrated in the prostate[42] and appeared to sensitise the prostate to the action of androgen[43] and also to ACTH acting via the adrenals[44]. Pituitary prolactin output had been shown experimentally to increase after total prostatectomy and castration in rats and to be suppressed by crude extract of prostate[45].

Several methods have been used to destroy the pituitary, including surgical ablation, irradiation by external sources or by implantation of radioactive materials, cryosurgery, thermo-coagulation and ultrasound. Complete destruction has gener-ally been uncommon, but there seems to be good evidence that this is not necessary to achieve useful clinical remission.

SURGICAL HYPOPHYSECTOMY

Surgical hypophysectomy has usually been done using a right or left frontal or fronto-temporal approach. Satisfactory exposure is then obtained by retraction of the frontal lobe, except for the occasional patient with a prefixed optic chiasma, or when the frontal lobe contains metastases. The pituitary stalk is divided and the gland removed in pieces by curettage, abrasive swabbing and suction, until the fossa is emptied as thoroughly as possible without provoking excessive bleeding. Particular care is usually taken to remove fragments lying anteriorly beneath the jugum sphenoidale. Any residual tissue may then be destroyed by application of Zenker's solution[46–48] or by local implantation of radioactive seeds[49]. Alternatively the trans-ethmosphenoidal approach has been used[50]; subse-quent leakage of cerebrospinal fluid occurred in only 32 of 258 cases and was controlled by packing the cavity with fascia lata and muscle.

Immediate mortality has varied following this procedure. Ray[51] recorded a series of 450 patients with metastatic breast or prostatic cancer, with an overall mortality within 30 days of only 6.7%. However, a higher mortality rate has generally been recorded with series confined to prostatic cancer, probably as a result of the older age of the patients. Luft and Olivecrona[48] in 1957 observed three early deaths in ten patients and more recently Murphy et al.[52] described an immediate mortality of two of eleven patients (18.2%).

Urinary gonadotrophins and ACTH are profoundly depressed following surgical hypophysectomy and the majority of patients show depression of thyroid function[47,52]. The most sensitive endocrine test for residual pituitary tissue is the human growth hormone (HGH) response to insulin induced hypoglycemia. West and Murphy[54] have shown an absence of response in all eight patients who underwent open hypo-physectomy (mean pre-operative levels 15.6 ± 0.8 ng/ml of plasma, compared to levels of 0.94 ± 0.03 post-operatively, expressed as integrated average growth hormone level during a 90 min period). It will be seen in succeeding sections that this index of pituitary function is less reliably suppressed by other methods of ablation.

The completeness of pituitary removal by surgery has been assessed anatomically by Pearson and Ray[47], who removed the entire sella turcica at autopsy in 35 cases, decalcified the specimens and then made serial sections. In 21 cases (60%) there was no residual pituitary tissue; in a further ten (28.5%) there were small microscopic foci only, representing less than 2% of the original pituitary mass; in four (11.5%) there was gross residue, which amounted to less than 10% in three cases; however in one case almost the whole gland was still present—interestingly, this patient enjoyed a good objective remission lasting seven months.

Some clinical results of surgical hypophysectomy in patients with prostatic cancer are summarised in Table 7.2. In general, rather more than half of the patients who survived the procedure experienced subjective improvement in their symptoms and in many of these cases good objective evidence of tumor regression was described. Pain relief was usually achieved within a week of the operation[49] and the average duration of remission in eight cases described by West and Murphy[54] was 6.78 ± 2.26 months. Some patients survived for over two years after this procedure[48] and good response was described in two cases who had failed to respond to previous endocrine therapy[48].

Table 7.2 SUMMARY OF SOME REPORTED RESULTS OF SURGICAL HYPOPHYSECTOMY IN PATIENTS WITH PROSTATIC CANCER

Author and year (Ref.)	Number of cases	Early deaths	Improvement Subjective	Objective
Scott[11]	6	2	2	2
Pearson et al.[46]	4	—	1	1
Luft and Olivecrona[48]	10	3	5	—
Smith et al.[49]	5	1	4	4
Ray[51]	16	—	6	—
Scott and Schirmer[12]	17	3	7/10	7/10
Murphy et al.[52]	11	2	7	—

STEREOTAXIC CRYOHYPOPHYSECTOMY

This method of destruction of the pituitary was introduced by Wilson *et al.*[55] in 1966 and has been extensively evaluated by Norrell and colleagues[56,57] and by Murphy and colleagues[52-54]. This procedure has been performed under local anesthetic, with the head held in a stereotactic frame. The midline of the anterior-inferior quadrant of the sella turcica was taken as target point and its position verified by collimated X-ray films in two planes. A twist drill was passed through the nose, avoiding the turbinate if possible; the anterior wall of the sphenoid sinus was penetrated and a single opening made through the anterior wall of the sella turcica and through the dural lining without passing more than 1–2 mm into the pituitary gland. A 4.2 mm cryoprobe (Linde) was then positioned at the target point and a single midline lesion created with the probe at − 186 °C for 15 min. During freezing, the visual fields and extraocular muscle activity was examined frequently. The probe was then thawed and removed. If rhinorrhea persisted for more than two weeks, the sphenoid sinus was packed with thigh muscle.

The nature and extent of the pituitary destruction was established by pathological examination of the entire sphenoid bone including the sella turcica by decalcification and serial sectioning[56]. The defect in the sphenoid was initially plugged by fibrin, which was later replaced by fibrous tissue. Within the first month of cryosurgery, extensive coagulation necrosis and hemorrhagic infarction was found throughout the anterior lobe. Any residual viable anterior pituitary tissue was invariably found on a lateral border of the gland, adjacent to the cavernous sinus and carotid artery. After four months, the damaged area had been replaced by collagenous scar tissue. In no case was total destruction achieved. No carotid artery damage was found, but extensive fibrosis and axonal degeneration in the oculomotor nerve was observed in one case.

The extent of the destruction was correlated in 18 cases with the change in hormone measurements observed during life, which included measurement of gonadotrophins, TSH, ACTH and HGH[56]. All of these variables were depressed in four cases in which less than 1% of the original pituitary mass remained. With more than 3% residual pituitary, detectable levels of growth hormone were usually found, but TSH and ACTH did not generally appear except for one case in which 28% residual tissue was present. Gonadotrophin was only found in one case with 49% residual pituitary.

In this series of 60 patients of both sexes, Norrell et al.[56] reported that six cases (10%) died within one month. Persistent rhinorrhea occurred in six cases (10%) but had not occurred in the most recent 40 patients. Persistent diabetes insipidus occurred in six cases (10%). The clinical results achieved by these workers with 20 patients with metastatic prostatic cancer were described by Maddy et al.[57]. Overall, 12 patients (63%) achieved a remission that lasted for three months or longer: in seven cases both subjective and objective evidence of regression was found and the other five showed subjective improvement with decrease in pain, weight gain and improvement in blood count and appetite. Average survival for patients showing a good response was 11.5 months and for non-responders 3.8 months. Response was not related to age or duration of disease and one-third of patients who had failed to respond to previous endocrine therapy showed a response to pituitary ablation. Objective evidence of response was seen irrespective of the precise degree of pituitary destruction and even occurred in the case with 49% residual tissue.

Murphy et al.[52] found that although cryosurgery was safer than open craniotomy, the results were inferior. Only five of twenty-three patients (21.7%) treated by cryosurgery achieved a satisfactory remission, as compared to seven of eleven (63.3%) with open craniotomy. The extent of pituitary destruction was graded on the basis of the growth hormone response to insulin induced hypoglycemia[52,54] and a "percentage index of ablation" was calculated: eight open craniotomy cases showed an average of 93.9% ablation; cryosurgery cases were divided into maximal ablation (seven cases—90.3%); intermediate (five cases—73.3%); and minimal (seven cases— average 22.2% ablation). No patients with minimal inhibition of pituitary function showed improvement, but a similar percentage (42.9 and 40.0%) of cases in the groups with intermediate or maximal pituitary inhibition showed a satisfactory remission. Survival was significantly longer (average 13.58 and 13.57 months) in patients in groups with intermediate or maximal pituitary inhibition, as compared to those with minimal ablation (average 4.80 months). It was concluded that effective pituitary ablation significantly improved the length of survival and duration of remission, compared to cases with non-effective ablation.

Murphy et al.[52] also observed that plasma testosterone was slightly but not significantly lower in responders (18.3 ± 3.48) as compared to non-responders (50.66 ± 23.06 ng/100 ml) at three months after pituitary destruction, but this difference was not apparent at six months. Urinary 17-ketosteroids were slightly lower at three months in responders compared with non-responders, but this difference appeared to be due more to the non-androgenic (11-oxy-) fraction, than to the andro-genic 11-deoxy-17-ketosteroids.

Farnsworth[58] observed dramatic relief of severe pain from bone metastases following this procedure in three of four patients, but felt that this improvement was not accompanied by any postponement of death from tumor progression.

RADIOFREQUENCY HYPOPHYSECTOMY

Zervas and Gordy[59] used a bilateral stereotaxic technique to introduce insulated 2.1 mm electrodes (with 5 mm uninsulated tips) and a thermistor probe into the pituitary fossa. With very high frequency (1–2 megacycles) currents, controlled heating of the tissues was obtained. Unipolar currents were applied to each side for 5 min and then a bipolar current for 10 min, which raised the pituitary temperature to 80 °C. Eleven patients with prostatic cancer were treated: two showed objective evidence of tumor regression, with healing of bone metastases and survival for 8 and 18 months; a further four cases became painfree and the remaining five patients did not respond and were dead within five months.

PITUITARY IRRADIATION

The anterior part of the normal pituitary is extremely radio-resistant. It has been calculated[60,61] that 100 000–200 000 rads are required to destroy it. It is therefore not surprising that attempts to irradiate the normal pituitary with con-ventional external radiotherapy equipment have met with little success[62]. More success has been achieved by Lawrence and colleagues with proton irradiation from a 340 MeV generator, giving 24–30 000 rads by a multiplane, rotational technique[63], or with high energy α particles, protons or deuterons generated by a 184 inch cyclotron, using either rotation techniques or the Bragg curve peak effect[64]. A degree of pituitary suppression was achieved in 146 women with advanced breast carcinoma, but cranial nerve damage or temporal lobe injury leading to temporal lobe seizures occurred in eleven patients and evidence of radiation damage to adjacent structures was found in more cases at autopsy. Experimental work with heavy particle irradiation is continuing, but for the destruction of the normal pituitary, local implantation of a radioactive source has been found easier and more useful in clinical practice.

In 1934, Lacassagne and Nyka[65] showed that the rabbit pituitary could be destroyed by radon seeds introduced with a fine needle. Initial attempts to use an orbital approach failed and eventually a transfrontal approach was used. Little progress was made until the stereotaxic pernasal trans-phenoidal route was defined by Talairach et al.[66] in 1956.

Initially, various radioactive materials were used and their physical characteristics and effects on the pituitary and adjacent structures have been admirably summarised by Forrest et al.[67]. Radon seeds produce penetrating γ rays (maximum energy 1.8 MeV) and irreparable damage to the optic chiasma was produced in eight of twelve patients with advanced breast cancer who survived more than six months; complete pituitary destruction was found in only one of twenty patients. Radioactive gold (^{198}Au) emits both β particles and γ rays (maximum energy of β particles 0.96 MeV and of γ rays, 0.41 MeV). Its equivalent activity in terms of γ irradiation dose is approximately one-fifth that of radon (1 mCi radon = 4.8 mCi ^{198}Au). Fergusson used ^{198}Au screened gold grains (3.8–9.0 mCi) and unscreened gold rods (0.8–4.57 mCi) in nine patients with advanced prostatic cancer and the effects on the pituitary were described by Young[68]. A radius of necrosis of 0.9–3.34 mm was achieved, but it was estimated that γ radiation produced a dose of 68 000–93 000 rads at the edge of the area of necrosis and some damage to optic nerves was observed.

Yttrium 90 was introduced as a β particle source for pituitary destruction by Rasmussen and colleagues[60] in 1953. Yttrium 89 is the only natural isotope of this element and it absorbs one neutron to become Yttrium 90. This then decays to Zirconium 90, a stable isotope, by emitting a β particle with a maximum energy of 2.3 MeV. It has a half-life of 62 hours, so that it reaches nearly 90% of saturation activity after one week in the atomic pile. The tissue dose falls off by a factor of 10 for each 2 mm of distance from the source and the maximum range in soft tissues is only about 1 cm. Thus a well-placed source of the correct dosage should not irradiate the optic chiasma, which would only be at risk if the rod was placed too high in the upper half of the fossa. The rods are produced by mixing finely powdered pure yttrium oxide (Y_2O_3) with a DPX mountant, which is then compressed into a thick-walled capillary tube. The rods are then extruded and dried, before being transferred to a crucible. Firing then takes place in stages, ending in a high frequency generator at 1650–1700 °C. The sintering which occurs produces rods which are strong enough to handle and these are cut to an appropriate size (1.3 × 3.95 mm—Fergusson[69]; 2.3 × 6.3 mm—Forrest[67]). When required for use, they are dispatched for activation in the atomic pile and generally have an activity of 3 to 5 mCi per rod when they reach the hospital.

The radio-active yttrium is inserted per-nasally either as rods or encased in a nylon sheath as screws. The technique of insertion of the rods has been described in detail by Fergusson[69]. The rods are supplied in a cylindrical cartridge for loading into the breech of the introducing needle. Two stilettes are provided, one with a sharp point to occlude the lumen of the needle during its introduction into the pituitary and the other to eject the radioactive rod from the cartridge and on through the needle. A preliminary X-ray of skull is taken to check the relative positions of the pituitary fossa and clinoid processes. Under general anesthetic, the head is placed precisely vertically on a supporting wooden block and the preliminary cocaine and adrenaline pack is removed from the nose. The needle is then introduced into the nose, avoiding the turbinates, until the anterior wall of the sphenoid sinus is reached. The position of the needle is then checked fluoroscopically in anterior and lateral planes and any necessary adjustments in position made. A light hammer tap takes the needle through the anterior wall of the sphenoid sinus and it then passes easily to reach the anterior wall of the pituitary fossa. The position is then checked again and further adjustments in position made so that the needle will enter the fossa low down close to the midline. A few more light hammer taps then carry the needle forward until it enters the pituitary fossa. The position is checked again, and the stilette is then withdrawn and the yttrium rod is inserted into the fossa. The procedure is then repeated on the other side and check films are taken (Figures 7.1 and 7.2). This procedure takes no more than 20–30 min and Fergusson has continued to use this simple method in over 100 cases.

Forrest et al.[67] used a similar method in their first 53 patients with breast cancer, giving a total dose of 8–17 mCi. Only five patients experienced visual disturbances, which were minimal in four and showed no tendency to progress, which had been a most undesirable feature with radon. The extent of pituitary destruction was assessed at autopsy in 23 cases: in four (11.2–13.0 mCi) destruction was complete; in eleven (10.0–16.0 mCi) 90–99% complete; and in six (8.5–15 mCi) only 50–80% destruction was achieved (two patients died within 24 hours and showed 0–30% destruction). The variation in destruction appeared to correlate with the variable position of the yttrium rods and Forrest et al.[70] therefore developed a 5 × 2 mm screw in which the yttrium rod was encased in a sharp-pointed nylon sheath; this was fitted into one end of a stainless steel self tapping orthopedic screw, the other end of which was turned down and screwed with a 6 BA die. The pituitary fossa was entered with a preliminary drill hole and the yttrium screw was then inserted, with a special screwdriver and held precisely in the desired position by the screw threading into the bone, which also served to close the defect in the anterior wall of the pituitary fossa. Twelve cases were examined at post-mortem (12.6–14.5 mCi total dose) and 98–100% destruction was found in all cases.

The total dose of irradiation given by Forrest et al.[67] was 13.8–14.5 mCi in the first 33 cases using the yttrium screws, but two patients developed visual defects and diabetes insipidus was seen in all cases who received over 14 mCi. The dose was

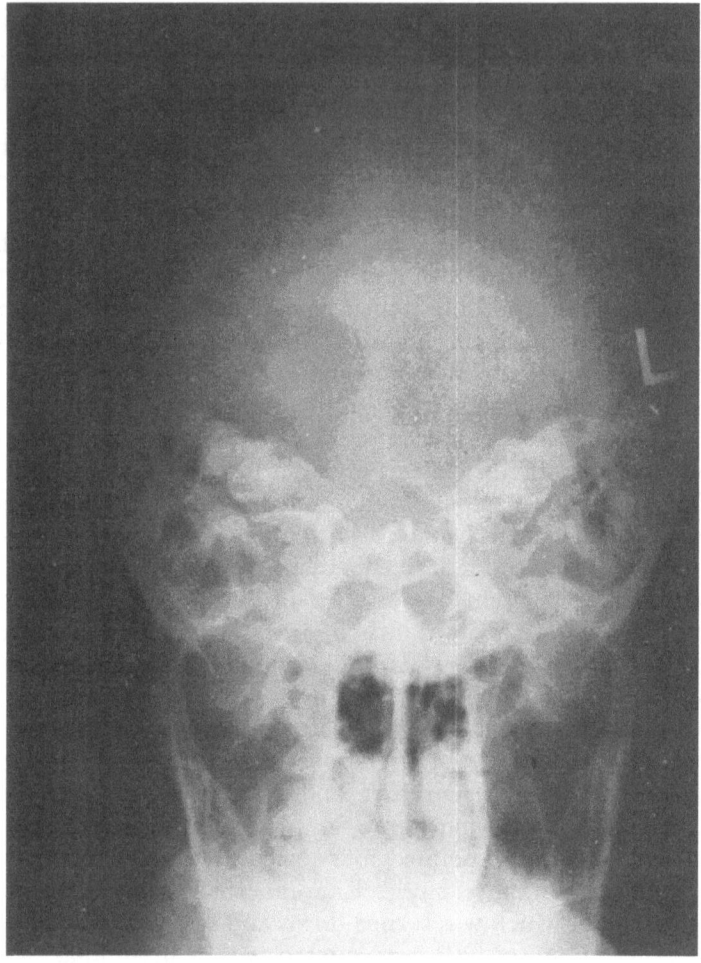

therefore reduced to 9.0–9.2 mCi in six cases and no complications were observed, although pituitary destruction appeared
to be equally satisfactory. Similarly Fergusson initially used
three rods of about 4 mCi, but now uses only two, with equally
good clinical response and very few adverse side effects.

The pathological changes occurring after pituitary ablation with yttrium 90 have been described by Kelly et al.[61], in
19 specimens obtained from 20 hours to 16 months after
implantation. In the first 24 hours, edema, vascular thrombosis

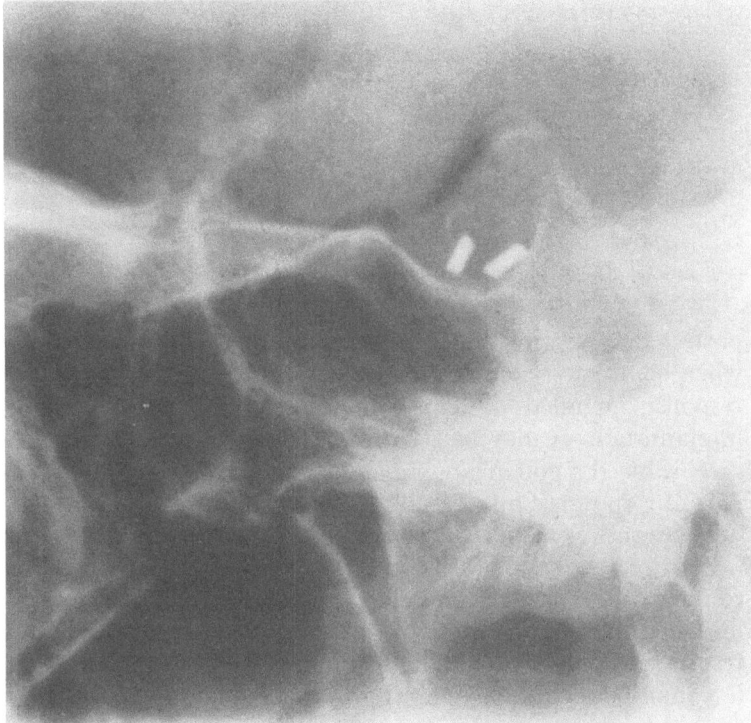

Figures 7.1 and 7.2   Antero-posterior and lateral views of two yttrium 90 rods after implantation by the needle technique; note that both needles are situated near the midline, in the lower half of the pituitary fossa

and tissue disruption from trauma were noted. By five days, extensive central necrosis was found, with edema, hemorrhage and early phagocytosis. By nine days a clear-cut edge had appeared, but degenerative changes were seen for up to two months after implantation. Chromophobe, eosinophil and basophil cells appeared to be equally sensitive[61,68].

The subjective clinical response in patients with advanced prostatic cancer is summarised from five published reports in Table 7.3. The response was graded as good when metastatic pain, or the symptom complex resulting from some major complication such as paraplegia or bladder neck obstruction was relieved completely and relief continued until death or only shortly before. Cases were said to have responded when

Table 7.3 SOME CLINICAL RESULTS OF PITUITARY IRRADIATION WITH YTTRIUM 90

Author and year (Ref.)	Number of cases	Response to implantation		
		Good	Responded	No response
Bennett and Harris[71]	2	1	—	1
Sedan and Harter[72]	14	8 (57%)	3 (21.5%)	3 (21.5%)
Straffon et al.[73]	13	7 (54%)	4 (31%)	2 (15%)
Morales et al.[74]	23	12 (52%)	6 (26%)	5 (22%)
Fergusson and Hendry[75]	100	39 (%)	32 (%)	29 (%)

partial but worthwhile relief of symptoms was achieved, or when complete relief was followed by subsequent relapse. No response included patients who died within one month of implantation. It may be seen from Table 7.3 that 39–57% of cases showed a good response and a further 20–31% showed a partial response. Only 15–29% showed no response at all.

Fergusson and Hendry[75] analysed the results in 100 cases in relation to several other factors and showed that the previous response to estrogens or castration appeared to have little influence on the subsequent result of implantation. A favorable response appeared to be slightly more likely in patients aged less than 60, or in patients who had had the disease for more than three years. In this series diabetes insipidus occurred in 22 of 100 cases and responded quickly to treatment with Pituitrin snuff or Pitressin tannate. Six patients early in the series showed evidence of cranial nerve damage. Two patients showed visual field defects and one patient went blind in one eye following a second implantation for recurrence of pain, two years and ten months after the first successful treatment. Three ocular palsies occurred. Slight leakage of cerebrospinal fluid occurred in 25 cases, but in only four cases did this persist for more than a few days. It ultimately dried up in all patients except one, who underwent successful trans-ethmoidal/sphenoidal exploration nine months after implantation. Four patients died of meningitis early in the series; a further four patients showed signs of meningitis in the second 50 cases, all of whom recovered with antibiotic therapy. It is our present practice to give ampicillin routinely before and for a few days after operation and this complication has not been encountered recently. Three patients developed hemiplegia and died within three weeks of implantation. Although this had not previously been recognised as a complication of this procedure, radiation damage to the cavernous portions of the internal carotid arteries has been described in six cases[76].

Serial studies in seven patients showed a marked drop in plasma testosterone within one week of pituitary ablation, which rose gradually over the next three months, but remained on average slightly below pre-implantation levels[77]. Other studies have shown rapid reduction in urinary gonadotrophin levels after implantation, even though Metapirone stimulation showed some residual pituitary activity by growth hormone assay[78,79].

Many authors have commented on the rapidity with which bone pain disappears after this procedure, which Sedan and Harter[72] described as "d'une façon spectaculaire et dès le lendemain de l'implantation".

Roberts *et al.*[80] have compared the results of yttrium 90 implantation with surgical transethmoidal hypophysectomy in 100 patients with advanced breast carcinoma in a controlled clinical trial. The remission rate, length of survival and depression of pituitary function as assessed by growth hormone response to stimulation were similar in both groups and it was concluded that there was no significant difference between the results achieved by these two techniques. In a further controlled trial[81] it was shown that there was no advantage in performing pituitary ablation early in the course of the disease and in some cases it may even have done harm.

Brendler[82] has concluded that this procedure should be reserved for selected patients who have relapsed after, or who are refractory to, conventional endocrine therapy. There seems little doubt that it can then form a valuable part of the sequential management of the disease, the principles of which have been clearly defined by Fergusson[83].

REPLACEMENT THERAPY

After pituitary ablation by yttrium 90 implantation, replacement therapy should be started the next day with cortisone acetate 25 mg twice daily by mouth, and in most cases this can be reduced to 37.5 mg daily after 7–10 days. Any subsequent severe stress or operation is covered by hydrocortisone (100 mg i.m. given before and 6-hourly after operation, reducing by steps until the original maintenance dose is reached). Diabetes insipidus may develop in 10–20% of cases, and usually responds quickly to Pituitrin snuff, the dose of which is adjusted to control the symptoms. Clinical evidence of myxedema is uncommon, but Norrell et al.[56] have shown that if protein-bound iodine and ^{131}I uptake are below normal at six weeks, the levels are likely to remain depressed throughout the remainder of the patient's survival. If clinical signs of myxedema develop, replacement therapy with thyroxin 0.1–0.3 mg/day should be given.

Summary and conclusions

This survey has provided ample evidence that suppression of adrenal or pituitary function can make the final months of life more comfortable for many patients with disseminated metastases from carcinoma of the prostate. Bilateral adrenalectomy is probably an unnecessarily severe surgical procedure, but a good though short-lived response can sometimes be obtained by adrenal suppression with cortisone. Pituitary ablation appears to give more consistently satisfactory results and of the methods available at present, irradiation by Yttrium 90 implantation is probably the safest and most reliable technique.

REFERENCES

1. Huggins, C., Stevens, R. E. and Hodges, C. V. (1941). Studies on prostatic cancer. II. The effects of castration on advanced carcinoma of the prostate gland. *Arch. Surg.*, *43*, 209

2. Huggins, C. and Hodges, C. V. (1941). Studies on prostatic cancer. I. Effect of castration, of estrogen, and of androgen injection on serum phosphatases in metastatic carcinoma of the prostate. *Cancer Res.*, *1*, 293

3. Scott, W. W. and Vermuelen, C. (1942). Studies on prostatic cancer. Excretion of 17-ketosteroids, estrogens and gonadotrophins before and after castration. *J. Clin. Endocrinol.*, *2*, 450

4. Dean, A. L., Woodard, H. Q. and Twombley, G. H. (1944). The endocrine treatment of cancers of the prostate gland. *Surgery*, *16*, 169

5. Huggins, C. and Scott, W. W. (1945). Bilateral adrenalectomy in prostatic cancer: clinical features and urinary excretion of ketosteroids and estrogen. *Ann. Surg.*, *122*, 1031

6. Cox, H. T. (1947). Adrenalectomy and prostatic cancer. *Lancet, ii*, 425

7. Thorn, G. W., Forsham, P. H., Frawley, T. F., Hill, S. R., Roche, M., Staehelin, D. and Wilson, D. L. (1950). The clinical usefulness of ACTH and cortisone. *New Engl. J. Med.*, *242*, 783

8. Huggins, C. and Bergenstal, D. M. (1951). Surgery of the Adrenals. *J. Amer. Med. Ass.*, *147*, 101

9. Scott, W. W. (1952). Endocrine management of disseminated prostatic cancer, including bilateral adrenalectomy and hypophysectomy. *Trans. Amer. Ass. Gen.-Urin. Surg.*, *44*, 101

10. Scott, W. W. (1953). Appraisal of present methods of treatment of advanced prostatic cancer. *Trans. Amer. Ass. Gen.-Urin. Surg.*, *45*, 39

11. Scott, W. W. (1954). Role of pituitary in normal and abnormal prostatic growth. *Trans. Amer. Ass. Gen.-Urin. Surg.*, *46*, 33

12. Scott, W. W. and Schirmer, H. K. A. (1962). Hypophysectomy for disseminated prostatic cancer. In *On Cancer and Hormones*, p. 175. (Chicago: University of Chicago Press.) Quoted by Brendler[82]

13. Grayhack, J. T., Bunce, P. L., Kearns, J. W. and Scott, W. W. (1955). Influence of the pituitary on prostatic response to androgen in the rat. *Bull. Johns Hopk. Hosp.*, *96*, 154

14. Morales, P. A., Brendler, H. and Hotchkiss, R. (1955). Role of adrenal cortex in prostatic cancer. *J. Urol.*, *73*, 399

15. Schoonees, R., Schalch, D. S., Reynoso, G. and Murphy, G. P. (1972). Bilateral adrenalectomy for advanced prostatic carcinoma. *J. Urol.*, *108*, 123

16. Pyrah, L. N. (1956). Hormones in the treatment of cancer of the breast and prostate; with special reference to the adrenal gland. *Brit. J. Surg.*, *44*, 69

17. Macfarlane, D. A., Thomas, L. P. and Harrison, J. H. (1960). A survey of total adrenalectomy in cancer of the prostate. *Amer. J. Surg.*, *99*, 562

18. Huggins, C. and Bergenstal, D. M. (1952). Inhibition of human mammary and prostatic cancer by adrenalectomy. *Cancer Res.*, *12*, 134

19. Mahoney, E. M. and Harrison, J. H. (1972). Bilateral adrenalectomy for palliative treatment of prostatic cancer. *J. Urol.*, *108*, 936

20. Scardino, P. L., Prince, C. L. and McGoldrick, T. A. (1953). Bilateral adrenalectomy for prostatic cancer. *J. Urol.*, *70*, 100

21. Young, H. H. (1936). A technique for simultaneous exposure and operation on the adrenals. *Surg. Gynecol. Obstet.*, *63*, 179

22. Thorn, G. W., Jenkies, D., Laidlaw, J. C., Goetz, F. C., Dingman, J. F., Arons, N. C., Streeten, D. H. P. and McCracken, B. H. (1953). Medical progress: pharmacologic aspects of adrenocortical steroids and ACTH in man. *New Engl. J. Med.*, *248*, 632

23. Hollander, V. P., West, C. D., Whitmore, W. F., Randall, H. T. and Pearson, O. H. (1952). Physiological effects of bilateral adrenalectomy in man. *Cancer, 5*, 1019

24. Munson, P. L., Goetz, F. C., Laidlaw, J. C., Harrison, J. H. and Thorn, G. W. (1954). Effect of adrenocortical steroids on androgen excretion by adrenalectomized orchidectomised men. *J. Clin. Endocrinol.*, *14*, 495

25. West, C. D., Hollander, V. P., Whitmore, W. F., Randall, H. T. and Pearson, O. H. (1952). The effect of bilateral adrenalectomy upon neoplastic disease in man. *Cancer, 5*, 1009

26. Baker, W. J. (1953). Bilateral adrenalectomy for carcinoma of the prostate gland: preliminary report. *J. Urol.*, *70*, 275

27. Baker, W. J. (1954). Late results of bilateral adrenalectomy for advanced carcinoma of the prostate gland. *Trans. Amer. Ass. Gen.-Urin. Surg.*, *45*, 43

28. Butler, W. W. S., Grayhack, J. T., Ransom, C. L. and Scott, W. W. (1953). Metabolic studies on the bilateral adrenalectomy patient. *J. Urol.*, *70*, 657

29. Harrison, J. H., Thorn, G. W., Jenkins, D. (1953). Total adrenalectomy for reactivated carcinoma of the prostate. *New Engl. J. Med.*, *248*, 86

30. Birke, G., Franksson, C. and Plantin, L. O. (1955). Steroid response to hormone therapy in prostatic cancer. *Acta Chir. Scand.*, *109*, 129

31. Fergusson, J. D. (1958). Endocrine-control therapy in prostatic cancer. *Brit. J. Urol.*, *30*, 397

32. Franks, L. M. (1953). Structural changes in prostatic cancer after bilateral adrenalectomy. *Brit. Med. J.*, *2*, 359

33. Harrison, J. H., Leman, C. B., Munson, P. L. and Laidlaw, J. C. (1955). Androgen, gonadotropin, and steroid excretion in man before and after castration and adrenalectomy. *J. Urol.*, *73*, 580

34. Burt, F. B., Finney, R. P. and Scott, W. W. (1957). Steroid response to hormone therapy in prostatic cancer. *Cancer*, *10*, 825

35. Pearson, O. H., Whitmore, W. F., West, C. D., Farrow, J. H. and Randall, H. T. Clinical and metabolic studies of bilateral adrenalectomy. *Surgery*, *34*, 543

36. Whitmore, W. F. (1956). Hormone therapy in prostatic cancer. *Amer. J. Med.*, *21*, 697

37. Ray, E. H. (1957). Endocrine therapy of prostatic carcinoma. *J. Amer. Med. Ass.*, *163*, 1008

38. Reynoso, G. and Murphy, G. P. (1972). Adrenalectomy and hypophysectomy in advanced prostatic carcinoma. *Cancer*, *29*, 941

39. Valk, W. L. and Owens, R. H. (1954). Endocrine inhibition as related to carcinoma of the prostate. *J. Urol.*, *72*, 516

40. Miller, G. M. and Hinman, F. (1954). Cortisone treatment in advanced carcinoma of the prostate. *J. Urol.*, *72*, 485

41. Robinson, M. R. G., Shearer, R. J. and Fergusson, J. D. (1974). Adrenal suppression in the treatment of carcinoma of prostate. *Brit. J. Urol.* (in press)

42. Sonnenberg, M., Money, W. L. and Rawson, R. W. (1954). Localization of radioactivity in the rat prostate after the administration of labeled prolactin preparations. *J. Clin. Endocrinol.*, *14*, 832

43. Segaloff, A., Steelman, S. L. and Flores, A. (1956). Prolactin as a factor in the ventral prostate assay for luteinizing hormone. *Endocrinology*, *59*, 233

44. Tullner, W. W. (1963). Hormonal factors in the adrenal-dependent growth of the rat ventral prostate. In *Biology of the Prostate and Related Tissues*, *12*, p. 211. (Bethesda, Maryland: National Cancer Institute Monograph)

45. Asano, M. (1965). Basic experimental studies of the pituitary prolactin-prostate interrelationships. *J. Urol.*, *93*, 87

46. Pearson, O. H., Ray, B. S., Harrold, C. C., West, C. D., Li, M. C., Maclean, J. P. and Lipsett, M. B. (1956). Hypophysectomy in treatment of advanced cancer. *J. Amer. Med. Ass.*, *161*, 17

47. Pearson, O. H. and Ray, B. S. (1960). Hypophysectomy in the treatment of metastatic mammary cancer. *Amer. J. Surg.*, *99*, 544

48. Luft, R. and Olivecrona, H. (1957). Hypophysectomy in the treatment of malignant tumours. *Cancer, 10,* 789
49. Smith, E. J. R., Gurling, K. J. and Baron, D. N. (1959). The effect of hypophysectomy in advanced cancer of prostate. *Brit. J. Urol., 31,* 181
50. Harrold, B. P., Cates, J. E. and James, J. A. (1968). Treatment of advanced cancer by trans-sphenoidal hypophysectomy. *Brit. J. Cancer, 22,* 19
51. Ray, B. S. (1960). Some inferences from hypophysectomy on 450 human patients. *Arch. Neurol., 3,* 121
52. Murphy, G. P., Reynoso, G., Schoonees, R., Gailani, S., Bourke, R., Kenny, G. M., Mirand, E. A. and Schalch, D. S. (1971). Hypophysectomy and adrenalectomy for disseminated prostatic carcinoma. *J. Urol., 105,* 817
53. Schoonees, R., Mittelman, A., Chheda, G. B. and Murphy, G. P. (1971). Urinary pseudouridine excretion following hypophysectomy for prostatic carcinoma in man. *J. Surg. Oncol., 3,* 25
54. West, C. R. and Murphy, G. P. (1973). Pituitary ablation and disseminated prostatic carcinoma. *J. Amer. Med. Ass., 225,* 253
55. Wilson, C. B., Winternitz, W. W., Bertan, V. and Sizemore, G. (1966). Stereotaxic cryosurgery of the pituitary gland in carcinoma of the breast and other disorders. *J. Amer. Med. Ass., 198,* 587
56. Norrell, H., Alves, A. M., Winternitz, W. W. and Maddy, J. (1970). A clinicopathologic analysis of cryohypophysectomy in patients with advanced cancer. *Cancer, 25,* 1050
57. Maddy, J. A., Winternitz, W. W. and Norrell, H. (1971). Cryohypophysectomy in the management of advanced prostatic cancer. *Cancer, 28,* 322
58. Farnsworth, R. H. (1972). Management of the terminal patient with prostatic cancer. *Brit. J. Urol., 44,* 122
59. Zervas, N. T. and Gordy, P. D. (1967). Radiofrequency hypophysectomy for metastatic breast and prostatic carcinoma. *Surg. Clin. N. Amer., 47,* 1279
60. Rasmussen, T., Harper, P. V. and Kennedy, T. (1953). The use of a Beta Ray Point source for destruction of the hypophysis. *Surgical Forum; Clinical Congress of the American College of Surgeons,* p. 681
61. Kelly, W. A., Evans, J. P., Harper, P. V. and Humphreys, E. M. (1958). The effect upon the hypophysis of radioactive yttrium. *Surg. Gynecol. Obstet., 106,* 600
62. Kelly, K. H., Fedsted, E. T., Brown, R. F., Ortega, P., Bierman, H. R., Low-Beer, B. V. and Shimkin, M. B. (1951). Irradiation of the normal human hypophysis in malignancy: Report of three cases receiving 8,000–10,000 r tissue dose to the pituitary gland. *J. Nat. Cancer Inst., 11,* 967
63. Lawrence, J. H. (1957). Proton irradiation of the pituitary. *Cancer, 10,* 795
64. Lawrence, J. H., Tobias, C. A., Born, J. L., Wang, C. C. and Linfoot, J. H. (1962). Heavy particle irradiation in neoplastic and neurologic diseases. *J. Neurosurg., 19,* 717
65. Lacassagne, A. and Nyka, W. (1934). Sur les processus histologiques de la destruction de l'hypophyse par le radon. *C.R. Soc. Biol. (Paris), 117,* 956
66. Talairach, J., Aboulker, J., Tournoux, P. and David, M. (1956). Technique stereotaxique de la chirurgie hypophysaire par voie nasale. *Neuro-chirurgerie, 2,* 3
67. Forrest, A. P. M., Blair, D. W., Peebles Brown, D. A., Stewart, H. J., Sandison, A. T., Harrington, R. W., Valentine, J. M. and Carter, P. T. (1959). Radioactive implantation of the pituitary. *Brit. J. Surg., 47,* 61

68. Young, S. Pituitary necrosis due to implants of radioactive gold and Yttrium. *Lancet, i,* 548

69. Fergusson, J. D. (1957). Implantation of radioactive material into the pituitary for the control of prostate cancer: an interium review. *Brit. J. Urol., 29,* 215

70. Forrest, A. P. M., Blair, D. W. and Valentine, J. M. (1958). Screw-implantation of the pituitary with Yttrium-90. *Lancet, ii,* 192

71. Bennett, R. C. and Harris, J. D. (1966). Pituitary ablation by implantation of Yttrium90 seeds. *Med. J. Aust., 2,* 673

72. Sedan, R. and Harter, M. (1966). Hypophysectomie dans les cancers de la prostate. *Neuro-chirugerie, 12,* 202

73. Straffon, R. A., Kiser, W. S., Robitaille, M. and Dohn, D. F. (1968). 90Yttrium hypophysectomy in the management of metastatic carcinoma of the prostate gland in 13 patients. *J. Urol., 99,* 102

74. Morales, A., Blair, D. W. and Steyn, J. (1971). Yttrium90 pituitary ablation in advanced carcinoma of the prostate. *Brit. J. Urol., 43,* 520

75. Fergusson, J. D. and Hendry, W. F. (1971). Pituitary irradiation in advanced carcinoma of the prostate: Analysis of 100 cases. *Brit. J. Urol., 43,* 514

76. Kaufman, B., Lapham, L. W., Shealy, C. N. and Pearson, O. H. (1966). Transphenoidal Yttrium 90 pituitary ablation: radiation damage to the internal carotid arteries. *Acta Radiol. Ther. Phys. Biol., 5,* 17

77. Shearer, R. J., Hendry, W. F., Sommerville, I. F. and Fergusson, J. D. (1973). Plasma testosterone: an accurate monitor of hormone treatment in prostatic cancer. *Brit. J. Urol., 45,* 668

78. Sprunt, J. G., Brownie, A. C. and Kinnear, J. S. (1963). Detection of incomplete ablation after Yttrium-90 implantation of pituitary. *Brit. Med. J., 2,* 1375

79. McCullagh, E. P., Feldstein, M. A., Tweed, D. C. and Dohn, D. F. (1965). A study of pituitary function after intrasellar implantation of 90Yttrium. *J. Clin. Endocrinol., 25,* 832

80. Roberts, M. M., Richards, S. H., Gleave, E. N., Stewart, H. J., Forrest, A. P. M., Joslin, C. A., Jones, V., Bouns, A. and Campbell, H. (1969). A controlled clinical trial to compare transethmoidal hypophysectomy with Yttrium implant of the pituitary in the treatment of advanced breast cancer. *Brit. J. Surg., 56,* 615

81. Stewart, H. J., Forrest, A. P. M., Roberts, M. M., Chinnock-Jones, R. E. A., Jones, V. and Campbell, H. (1969). Early pituitary implantation with Yttrium 90 for advanced breast cancer. *Lancet, ii,* 816

82. Brendler, H. (1973). Adrenalectomy and hypophysectomy for prostatic cancer. *Urology, 2,* 99

83. Fergusson, J. D. (1972). Sequential Management in Advanced Disease. In *Endocrine Therapy in Malignant Disease* (B. A. Stoll, editor) (London: Saunders)

Index